PORTLAND PRESS RESEARCH MONOGRAPH

Oxidative Stress, Lipoproteins and Cardiovascular Dysfunction

VII

PORTLAND PRESS RESEARCH MONOGRAPH VII

Oxidative Stress, Lipoproteins and Cardiovascular Dysfunction

Edited by
C. Rice-Evans
K.R. Bruckdorfer

PORTLAND PRESS

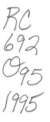

RC
692
O95
1995

#33242935   12-20-96

c.1

Published by Portland Press, 59 Portland Place, London W1N 3AJ, U.K.
In North America orders should be sent to Ashgate Publishing Co.,
Old Post Road, Brookfield, VT 05036-9704, U.S.A.

© 1995 Portland Press Ltd, London

ISBN 1 85578 045 3   ISSN 0964–5945

British Library Cataloguing in Publication Data
A catalogue record for this book is available from the British Library

Typeset and printed by Cambridge University Press, Cambridge

Contents

Preface

Over two decades ago, discussion of free radicals and antioxidants in relation to disease was regarded as a 'fringe' science. Today, entire conferences are devoted to the subject and attended by thousands. It is widely regarded as a legitimate part of the aetiology of a surprisingly large number of diseases. However, the area of cardiovascular research has now perhaps exceeded many of the others, in embracing the ideas of free radical biology to help explain many of the phenomena which have been so perplexing in the past. Nevertheless, much remains to be learned about how oxidation is initiated and about the roles of different lipids and lipoproteins fractions.

Oxygen presents a permanent challenge to vital processes because of its particular chemistry — its ability to produce a variety of reactive species [1]. Reactive oxygen species are formed as a consequence of normal metabolic processes and may be harnessed as part of the normal defence mechanism, e.g. by neutrophils and macrophages [2]. In consequence, all organisms have well-developed mechanisms to protect themselves against those forms of oxygen which have the potential to damage lipids, proteins and nucleic acids. Although dietary antioxidants form only part of this protection, they have attracted the greatest interest, particularly from the public, because of their obvious association with food, especially food deemed to promote good health.

During the 1970s, great strides were made in the understanding of the metabolism of cholesterol [3] and the establishment of this sterol as an important risk factor in vascular disease alongside smoking and hypertension, especially following the publication of the LRCS trial [4]. It should be made clear immediately that all discussion of lipoprotein oxidation, and the role of antioxidants in relation to cardiovascular disease, is an elaboration of the lipid hypothesis and not an alternative to it. Nevertheless, there are still unanswered questions concerning why some individuals have different clinical endpoints in a population with a high cholesterol profile, even taking into account the variation in smoking habits and hypertension. In this context, consumption of antioxidants may play a protective role, but is almost certainly not the sole explanation for all of this variation. In any case, their involvement may be linked with other factors such as smoking. There is increasing evidence that genetic factors, which regulate lipoprotein metabolism and that of other proteins related to cardio-vascular disease, may influence the impact of diet and other 'environ-mental' determinants of risk.

There are two principal developments which have led to the current interest in the reactive oxygen species and antioxidants in relation to cardiovascular disease. During the 1980s, considerable progress was made in the understanding of the chemistry of oxida-tion of lipoproteins (primarily the work of one of our authors, Professor Hermann Esterbauer, see Chapter 3) and the modification of certain amino acid residues on the apolipoproteins by aldehydes and other products of oxidation [5]. A bewildering number of prod-ucts are formed from cholesterol and from the fatty acids of chol-esterol esters and phospholipids, many of which are known to be cytotoxic. The other thrust came from the discovery by Professor Steinberg and co-workers that lipoproteins [particularly low-density lipoprotein (LDL)] may be oxidized by exposure to various cell types in culture [6]. From this and other work, a hypothesis was con-structed which included the oxidation of lipoproteins as an integral part of the development of atherosclerosis [7,8].

There are many differing views on the relative importance and timing of events which lead to the development of the athero-sclerotic plaque and the crucial events of thrombosis and vasospasm which follow from it. As in other disciplines, there are current fash-ions which cause the scientific community to leave their former inter-ests to pursue new developments which are perceived to be 'hot' at the time. In the 1970s, platelets were the topical interest to be superseded by new discoveries concerning the complexities of the endothelium and the potential consequences of early damage to endothelial function. The importance of smooth muscle proliferation was challenged by renewed interest in the role of macrophages, which are perceived to participate in the very earliest stage of the development of fatty streaks. Nevertheless, the fibrous cap resulting from the proliferative response often contributes most to the mass of the plaque. In this regard, the contributions by Professor Michael Davies and co-workers concerning the greater mechanical stability of plaques with thick fibrous caps, versus the more fragile lipid-rich plaques which are macrophage-rich, have been very illuminating [9].

The latter appear to pose the greatest danger because of their tendency to fissure and precipitate thrombotic episodes which lead to catastrophic clinical events. The debate concerning the supremacy of certain cell types in the artery wall in relation to atherogenesis has been shown to be somewhat sterile, in view of current understanding of the 'cross-talk' between them through the release of growth factors, interleukins, necrosis factors and many others [10]. The advances in the understanding of cell and molecular biology require an increasing sophistication of outlook and willingness to maintain an open mind.

Similar debates have occurred about the relative importance of different lipoprotein fractions, e.g. whether the plasma concentration of LDL is more important, or the various subfractions of the high-density lipoprotein fractions and the isoforms of some of the apolipoproteins found in the latter. In part, these divisions arise because of the limitations of what can be measured in blood samples in clinical laboratories, the processes occurring within the atherosclerotic plaque being less accessible. Lipoprotein(a) also attracted a great deal of interest and gave hope for some connection between the lipid school and those who believed that the coagulation system or fibrinolysis might be of greater importance in the clinical events in cardiovascular disease.

The perception of oxidative processes in relation to the current views on atherogenesis has been interesting. These ideas have appeared to unify a number of differing trends in the theories of atherogenesis which were mentioned above. The oxidation of lipoproteins appears to have an influence on a wide variety of cellular processes relevant to the development of atherosclerotic plaques and is outlined briefly below.

Following damage to the endothelium, or because of other signals, monocytes adhere to the endothelium, penetrate into the subendothelial region and become transformed into macrophages that express the scavenger receptor, which had previously been described for uptake of chemically modified LDL by macrophages. The LDL becomes slowly oxidized and is taken up by the macrophages which become stuffed with lipid, giving rise to the foam cells characteristic of atherosclerosis. Other modifications of LDL are possible, such as the formation of complexes with glycosaminogly-cans, which are taken up by a different mechanism [11]. The oxida-tion of the lipids yields products which modify many of the functions of cells in the artery wall which are exposed to them, e.g. enhancing the adhesion of monocytes to the endothelium and transforming monocytes into macrophages [12], exhibiting chemotactic properties which both attract further monocytes to the area and limit the egress of the macrophages from the artery wall [13]. Other effects of the oxidation products include the increased expression of tissue factor by the endothelium [14] and that of plasminogen activator inhibitor-1 [15], and diminution of endothelium-dependent relaxation of vascular smooth muscle induced by nitric oxide [16].

It is important to recognize that even mild oxidation of LDL (minimally modified LDL), where only small amounts of lipid are oxi-dized without discernible modification of the apolipoprotein, may produce some of the effects described above. At this level of oxida-tion, the LDL may not be completely toxic, but may modulate the transcriptional processes which lead to the synthesis of specific pro-teins by the cells. Oxidized LDL may also enhance the proliferative response of smooth muscle, leading to formation of the fibrous plaque.

The hypothesis that oxidized lipoproteins are involved in atherosclerosis was strengthened by the following observations. The presence of oxidized LDL in fresh human and animal atherosclerotic intima was demonstrated by the use of fluorescently labelled antibod-ies to epitopes on the modified apolipoprotein [18, 19]. There was cross-reactivity of antibodies to oxidized LDL with ceroid, commonly found in atherosclerotic tissue [20], suggesting that the latter may have originated from oxidized LDL. Auto-antibodies to oxidized LDL have been shown to exist in the circulation and that the titre is higher in patients with known cardiovascular disease [21]. It is generally thought that oxidized lipoproteins are found in the arterial intima and not in the plasma, since they would normally be removed rapidly from the circulation. However, loss into the circulation of some oxi-dized LDL may occur through the fissures in the atherosclerotic plaques, giving rise to the antibodies which have been found there. It is possible that mildly oxidized forms of the lipoproteins occur in the circulation, but this is still not certain. LDLs isolated from patients with known cardiovascular disease are more susceptible to oxidation, according to tests conducted in vitro by exposure to copper ions, compared with LDL from healthy controls [22, 23]. In experimental atherosclerosis, antioxidants such as probucol have been shown to inhibit strongly the progression, and enhance the regression, of atherosclerotic lesions [24].

The epidemiological evidence for a cardioprotective role for antioxidants is, however, still fragmentary and large-scale studies are still to be initiated and completed, which may take several years. There are still good grounds for advising the population as a whole to increase its dietary intake of fresh fruit and vegetables, since the benefits of this extend beyond a simple increase in antioxidants. The prescription of antioxidants is some way off, but it is likely that more members of the public and existing patients will take them anyway, as is already the case in the U.S.A. The description of the benefits of red wine in terms of its antioxidant qualities was no doubt welcome both to researchers and the public alike [23].

The role of reactive oxygen species in ischaemia–reperfusion injury has also attracted a great deal of interest. The technology employed for thrombolytic therapy of acute myocardial infarction gives rise to the problems caused by acute reoxygenation. Further difficulties may occur as a result of the widespread use of angioplasty. Both of these processes may give rise to restenosis through a rampant proliferative response accompanied by thrombosis. At least some of the processes described in relation to atherosclerosis are relevant here, and there is a clear interest in the role of free radicals in relation to tissue damage which is therefore encompassed in this book.

The aim of this book is to discuss the current understanding of the role of oxidative processes in atherosclerosis in terms of their chemistry, biochemistry and cell biology. It is not intended to be a treatise on the pathology of the process, although, among our contributors, there are individuals who are well qualified to do this. We have invited contributions from authors who are very active in this field. The aim was to bring together up-to-date information on current thinking in their respective fields and also to juxtapose differing perspectives of a common problem. For this we make no apology, because the mechanisms involved in these processes are not fully understood and comparisons of the views of leading workers in the field are of great value. Hopefully this will stimulate other workers, especially younger ones, to carry on this exciting work and to achieve even greater levels of understanding.

Catherine Rice-Evans
Richard Bruckdorfer
London 1994

References

1. Halliwell, B. and Gutteridge, J.M.C. (1985) in Free Radicals in Biology and Medicine, Clarendon Press, Oxford.
2. Babior, B.M. (1979) N. Engl. J. Med. **298**, 659–668
3. Brown, M.S. and Goldstein, J.L. (1986) Science **232**, 34–47
4. The Lipid Research Clinics Coronary Primary Prevention Trial Results: I. Reduction in the incidence of Coronary Heart Disease (1984) J. Am. Clin. Med. **251**, 351–364
5. Esterbauer, H., Dieber-Rotheneder, M., Waeg, G., Striegl, G. and Jurgens, G. (1990) Chem. Res. Toxicol. **3**, 77–91
6. Steinberg, D., Parthasarathy, S., Carew, T.E., Khoo, J.C. and Witztum, J.L. (1989) N. Engl. J. Med. **320**, 915–924
7. Steinberg, D. (1993) J. Intern. Med. **233**, 227–232
8. Rice-Evans, C. and Bruckdorfer, K.R. (1992) Free Radicals, Lipoproteins and Cardiovascular Dysfunction. Molecular Aspects of Medicine **13** (1), 1–111
9. Lendon, C.L., Davies, M.J. and Born, G.V.R. (1991) **87**, 87–99
10. Ross, R. (1993) Nature (London) **362**, 87–99
11. Vijayagopal, P., Srinivasan, S.R., Radhakrishnamurthy, B. and Berenson, G. (1993) Biochem. J. **289**, 837–844
12. Frostegard, J., Nilsson, J., Haegerstrand, A., Hamsten, A., Wigzell, H. and Gidlund, M. (1990) Proc. Natl. Acad. Sci. U.S.A. **87**, 904–908
13. Quinn, M.T., Parthasarathy, S., Fong, L.G. and Steinberg, D. (1987) Proc. Natl. Acad. Sci. U.S.A. **84**, 7725–7729
14. Drake, T.A., Hannani, K., Fei, H.H., Lavi, S. and Berliner, J.A. (1991) Am. J. Pathol. **138**, 601–607
15. Latron, Y., Chauton, M., Anforso, F., Alessi, M.C., Nalbone, G., Lafont, H. and Juhan-Vague, I. (1991) Arteriosclerosis Thrombosis 11, 1821–1829
16. Jacobs, M., Plane, F. and Bruckdorfer, K.R. (1990) Br. J. Pharmacol. **100**, 21–26
17. Yla-Herttuala, S., Palinski, W., Rosenfeld, M.E., Parthasarathy, S., Carew, T.E., Butler, S., Witztum, J.L. and Steinberg, D. (1989) J. Clin. Invest. **84,** 1086–1095
18. Rosenfeld, M.E., Palinski, W., Yla-Herttuala, S., Butler, S. and Witztum, J.L. (1990) Arteriosclerosis **10**, 336–349
19. Mitchinson, M.J., Ball, R.Y., Carpenter, K.L.H. and Parums, D.V. (1989) in Hyperlipidaemias and Atherosclerosis (Suckling, K.E. and Groot, P.E., eds.), pp. 117–134, Academic Press, London.
20. Salonen, J.T., Yla-Herttuala, S., Yamamoto, R., Butler, S., Korpela, H., Salonen, R., Nyyssonen, K., Palinski, W. and Witztum, J.L. (1992) Lancet **339**, 883–887
21. Davies, S.W., Datta, V.K., Balcon, R., Rice-Evans, C.A. and Bruckdorfer, K.R. (1991) Br. Heart. J. **66**, 78
22. Regnstrom, J., Nilsson, J., Tornvall, P., Landou, C. and Hamsten, A. (1992) Lancet **339**, 1183–1186

23. Nagano, Y., Nakamura, T., Matsuzawa, Y., Cho, M., Ueda, Y. and Kita, T. (1992) Atherosclerosis **93**, 131–140
24. Frankel, E.N., Kanner, J., German, J.B., Parks, E. and Kinsella, J.E. (1993) Lancet **341**, 454–457

Abbreviations

AAPH	2,2'-azo-bis-(2-amidinopropane)dihydrochloride
ACAT	acyl-CoA *O*-acyltransferase
ACh	acetylcholine
AMVN	2,2'-azo-bis-(2,4-dimethylvaleronitrile)
apo	apolipoprotein
CETP	cholesteryl ester transfer protein
CHD	coronary heart disease
CR-1	complement receptor-1
EDRF	endothelium-derived relaxing factor
EGF	epithelial growth factor
ELAM	endothelial leucocyte adhesion molecule
ETYA	eicosatetraynoic acid
FAD	flavin–adenine dinucleotide
FMN	flavin mononucleotide
GSH	reduced glutathione
HDL	high-density lipoprotein
5-HT	5-hydroxytryptamine
ICAM-1	intercellular adhesion molecule-1
IDL	intermediate-density lipoprotein
IFNγ	interferon γ
IL	interleukin
LCAT	lecithin–cholesterol acyltransferase
LDL	low-density lipoprotein
LO	lipoxygenase
Lp(a)	lipoprotein (a)
LRP	LDL-receptor-related protein
MAC	membrane attack complex
MCP	monocyte chemotactic protein
MPM	mouse peritoneal macrophages
NMDA	*N*-methyl-D-aspartate
NO	nitric oxide
NOS	nitric oxide synthase
oLDL	oxidized low-density lipoprotein
PAF	platelet activating factor

PBMC	peripheral blood mononuclear cells
PG	prostaglandin
PGH	prostaglandin endoperoxide
PGI$_2$	prostacyclin
PMA	phorbol 12-myristate 13-acetate
PMN	polymorphonuclear nucleocytes
PUFA	polyunsaturated fatty acid
SOD	superoxide dismutase
TBARS	thiobarbituric acid-reactive substances
TNF	tumour necrosis factor
VLDL	very low-density lipoprotein

Free radicals and antioxidants in normal and pathological processes

Catherine Rice-Evans

Free Radical Research Group, UMDS, Guy's Hospital, St Thomas's Street, London SE1 9RT, U.K.

Introduction

It is becoming well-recognized that reactive oxygen species such as superoxide and hydrogen peroxide may be important mediators of cell injury during disease processes via the oxidation of membranes or the alteration of critical enzyme systems.

Superoxide radicals and other active oxygen species are generated by a variety of cells in the body, through the action of oxidases and peroxidases etc., to perform useful functions. However, situations accompanying disease states may lead to enhanced superoxide radical production, over and above the requirements for normal metabolism, such as those involving excessive phagocyte activation, stimulation of the activity of enzymes such as xanthine oxidase, or disruption of mitochondrial electron transport. Thus, the availability in pathological states of excess active oxygen species, such as superoxide radical, hydrogen peroxide and hydroperoxides, may provide the direct production of potentially cytotoxic species. Once triggered, these processes may ultimately lead to modification of the activity of antioxidant enzymes through their inactivation or leakage from cells, or the release of metal ions from metalloproteins. Although superoxide radical is not very reactive *per se* it is the precursor of a number of reactive oxygen species: in its protonated form as the hydrogen dioxyl radical ($HO_2^{\cdot}$, pK_a 4.8) it can directly attack polyunsaturated fatty acids [1]; hydrogen peroxide, its dismutated form, easily diffuses through cell membranes; accumulation of hydroperoxides may arise through injury to tissues, activating phospholipases, cyclo-oxygenases and lipoxygenases; furthermore, peroxides generated by non-enzymic oxidation of polyunsaturated fatty acids or lipids can stimulate the action of cyclo-oxygenases and lipoxygenases, accelerating the production of prostaglandins and leukotrienes.

Fig. 1   **Mechanisms of amplification of superoxide reactivity by transition metals, haem proteins, nitric oxide or myeloperoxidase action**

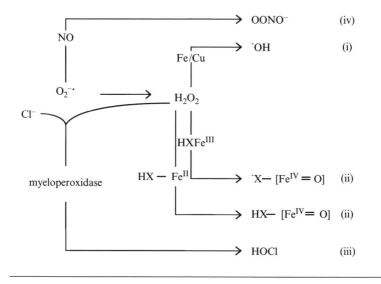

The reactivity of superoxide radical and hydrogen peroxide can be amplified (Fig. 1) by (i) reduction with available transition metal ions (iron or copper, if available) forming hydroxyl radicals; (ii) interaction with specific haem proteins (myoglobin or haemoglobin if available) inducing their activation to ferryl haem protein radicals; (iii) reaction with the myeloperoxidase released during the respiratory burst of neutrophils, forming hypochlorite, a very reactive oxidant which can damage proteins or further react to form long-lived chloramines; (iv) the reaction of superoxide with nitric oxide (NO), generating peroxynitrite anion which can oxidize a range of substrates. The possible decomposition of peroxynitrous acid to hydroxyl radical and the nitrogen dioxide radical has been proposed [2] and its relevance is discussed in Chapter 4 by Darley-Usmar and co-workers.

Injury to cells and tissues may also enhance the toxicity of the active oxygen species by releasing intracellular transition metal ions (such as iron) into the surrounding tissue from storage sites, decompartmentalized haem proteins, or metalloproteins by interaction with delocalized proteases or oxidants. Such delocalized iron and haem proteins have the capacity to decompose peroxide to peroxyl and alkoxyl radicals, exacerbating the initial lesion.

Thus the question arises as to what forms of haem protein and transition metal are available *in vivo* that are capable of mediating the formation of damaging initiating or propagating species. The majority of the iron and haem

Fig. 2 **Production of reactive oxygen species by phagocytic cells**

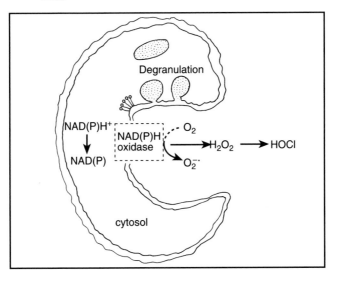

proteins in the human body are protected from exerting pro-oxidant activities by compartmentalization *in vivo* within their functional locations in the haem and non-haem iron-containing proteins and enzymes [3].

The 4 g of iron in the human body is normally compartmentalized into its functional locations in the haem- and non-haem-containing and iron-binding proteins and enzymes (Fig. 3). The majority (65%) of the iron is in the divalent state in haemoglobin and myoglobin, and is involved in the transport and storage of oxygen in erythrocytes and myocytes respectively. The rest is distributed between storage sites, predominantly in the liver, spleen and bone marrow, bound to ferritin, in the low-molecular-mass iron pool awaiting synthesis of iron-containing proteins and enzymes, or bound to transferrin (for transport) or lactoferrin. Transferrin is normally only 30% saturated, so any iron released into plasma will immediately be mopped up in the normal course of events.

Normally the only 'free' iron available is proposed to reside in the low-molecular-mass iron pool which is usually sequestered from exerting toxic effects. Trace transition metals or haem proteins may be redistributed or delocalized from their normal functional locations during cell damage. In some pathological situations, iron may be released from its normal functional compartments. Mobilization of iron from ferritin by superoxide radical, ascorbate and other reducing agents has been demonstrated [4–6]. This might occur in endothelial cells, which contain high levels of ferritin on generation of super-

Fig. 3   Normal body iron localization

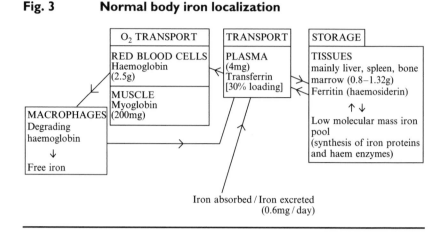

Iron absorbed / Iron excreted
(0.6mg / day)

oxide radicals at sites of damage, as observed in the inflamed rheumatoid joint, for example, or on reperfusion post-ischaemia.

Evidence is accumulating that when haemoglobin is released via microbleeding processes, it becomes toxic. Microbleeding has been observed in the eye, causing retinal damage [7], in the brain [8] and at sites of inflammation [9]. Immediately after an acute myocardial infarction there is an increase of myoglobin in the blood [10] on rupturing of cardiac myocytes. Increased local generation of hydrogen peroxide, formed from superoxide generation at the site of injury, may interact with delocalized myoglobin or haemoglobin. It has been shown in model systems *in vitro* that iron can be released from haemoglobin [11] and myoglobin [12,13] by excess hydrogen peroxide formed from superoxide radical, and from myoglobin by lipid hydroperoxides in oxidizing low-density lipoproteins (LDLs) [14]. This may be a mechanism for the availability of non-haem iron. The observed iron deposition in the artery wall in atherosclerotic lesions [15] may be the result of microbleeding from haemorrhaging in advanced lesions.

This question may be of considerable importance in the control of oxidation of LDLs in atherosclerosis and the potential mechanisms whereby LDL oxidation is amplified.

Sources of free radicals in normal physiological processes

Free radicals are essential to many physiological processes but can be highly destructive if produced in excess of normal requirements. In the human body, there is normally a balance between free radical (or pro-oxidant) production and antioxidant action. When the balance between pro-oxidants and antioxidants is tipped in favour of the former, the state of oxidative stress results [16]. In the normal course of events, free radicals participate in a number of biological events *in vivo*.

The action of oxidases: NADPH oxidase

Phagocytic cells produce superoxide radicals as part of their defence mechanisms. The cascade of events in the antimicrobial action of the phagocytic cells, neutrophils, monocytes, macrophages and eosinophils [17], occurs through the activity of the enzyme NADPH oxidase at the cell surface. Neutrophils are phagocytic cells which provide the first line of defence against invading microorganisms and are major contributors to the inflammatory response, accumulating at sites of inflammation where they act in a phagocytic or secretory capacity. Such phagocytic cells are activated when they encounter foreign particles, and undergo the respiratory burst essential for microbicidal activity. The cell flows around the bacterium or foreign particle and engulfs it within a plasma membrane vesicle or phagosome. Oxygen uptake in neutrophils and macrophages is thus due to the action of the NADPH oxidase complex associated with the plasma membrane (Fig. 2); the electrons released on oxidation of NADPH reduce oxygen to the superoxide radical (eqn. 1). The engulfed particles within the plasma membrane vesicle are therefore exposed to a high flux of superoxide radicals in the phagocyte cytoplasm, some of which are also released extracellularly. The importance of NADPH oxidase and the products of its action in the efficient killing of ingested bacteria is derived from observations of the consequences of its absence in chronic granulomatous disease, in which an extensive predisposition to severe and recurrent infection is characteristic [18].

The reaction products of superoxide ions may have a direct microbicidal effect [19], although, in view of its low reactivity, it is unlikely that superoxide itself is responsible for killing the invading material. The hydrogen peroxide formed from its dismutation (eqn. 2) can kill some strains of bacteria. Once the phagocytic vacuole is formed, fusion with other granules in the neutrophil cytoplasm releases myeloperoxidase which utilizes one of the products of the oxidase as a co-substrate with chloride, producing hypochlorite (eqns. 3–5) [20]. Hypochlorite can be involved in chloramine formation (eqn. 6). The following equations show the series of chemical events contributing towards bacterial killing.

$$2O_2 + NADPH \rightarrow 2O_2^{\cdot-} + NADP^+ + H^+ \tag{1}$$
$$2H^+ + 2O_2^{\cdot-} \rightarrow H_2O_2 + O_2 \tag{2}$$
$$MP^{3+} + H_2O_2 \rightarrow MP^{4+} = O + H^+ + OH^- \tag{3}$$
$$\underline{MP^{4+} = O + Cl^- \rightarrow MP^{3+} + OCl^- + H^+} \tag{4}$$

$$\text{Sum: } H_2O_2 + Cl^- \rightarrow HOCl + OH^- \tag{5}$$
$$OCl^- + RNH_2 \rightarrow RNHCl + OH \tag{6}$$

Superoxide may be protonated into the more reactive and cytotoxic hydrogen dioxyl radical (eqn. 7) in more acidic localities, such as the vacuole of the phagocyte or the microenvironment of cell membranes.

$$O_2^{-\cdot} + H^+ \rightarrow HO_2^{\cdot} \tag{7}$$

Thus, phagocytic cells produce a range of reactive oxygen species on activation, but there is no convincing evidence to suggest that these include the hydroxyl radical [21]. It is clear that through the reactions of superoxide anion and its products the phagosomal pH is increased, which is important for digestion of bacteria by proteinases [22,23]. Non-phagocytic cells, e.g. smooth muscle cells and endothelial cells, can also be stimulated to release superoxide by a range of mechanisms [24] (see below). Lymphocytes and fibroblasts [25–27] constantly generate small amounts of superoxide radical as possible growth regulators.

Chronic inflammatory disorders involve the generation of excessive levels of superoxide radicals: for example, adult respiratory distress syndrome, which is associated with excess phagocyte activation and neutrophil infiltration in the lungs; and joint disease with chronic persistent inflammation in the joints. It has been proposed that tissue damage may result from the stimulation of large numbers of phagocytes in a localized area. The local concentrations of oxidants formed by polymorphonuclear leucocytes can be extremely high. For example, experiments *in vitro* indicate that stimulation of 2×10^6 cells with 10 nM formylmethionylleucyl phenylalanine produces 10 nmol of superoxide per minute. In the absence of superoxide dismutase (SOD) and other superoxide-degrading pathways this would be a local concentration of 5–10 mM [28]. In the inflamed rheumatoid joint, chronic inflammation produces up to 500 nmol hydrogen peroxide per minute [29]. In reperfusion injury, the inflammatory response at sites of injury, on the endothelium, for example, after the ischaemic insult generates superoxide from activation of adherent neutrophils. This, in combination with intracellular sources of reactive oxygen species and the delocalization of haem proteins, may participate in tissue injury at the onset of reperfusion, which is additive to the tissue damage and secondary to the ischaemic insult.

Xanthine oxidase

Another potential source of oxygen-derived free radicals is the enzyme xanthine oxidase [30]. This enzyme is localized within the vascular endothelial cells. The conversion of xanthine dehydrogenase (which does not produce oxygen radicals) to xanthine oxidase (which produces superoxide and hydrogen peroxide) in response to inflammatory mediators has been reported [31]. During ischaemia, two major priming events for radical production have been proposed: namely catabolism of ATP to hypoxanthine and xanthine, and conversion of xanthine dehydrogenase to xanthine oxidase by a calcium-dependent protease activated by the increased calcium levels. The reintroduction of oxygen in relative excess at the time of reperfusion allows the xanthine oxidase-catalysed conversion of oxygen to superoxide and hydrogen peroxide [32]. The precise importance of xanthine oxidase in mechanisms of reperfusion injury in the human heart is still a matter of some debate.

In other organs, the endothelial cell-trigger mechanism based on xanthine oxidase is given a predominant role as a generator of superoxide in reperfusion injury (see Chapter 8). Direct evidence for the role of superoxide in reoxygenation injury has been derived from studies in which the reperfused feline ileum was protected *in vivo* by the systemic administration of SOD [33]. The fact that superoxide radical was a source of oxidative injury in post-ischaemic reoxygenation damage was implied by the protective role of allopurinol, an inhibitor of xanthine dehydrogenase and xanthine oxidase [34].

In a series of elegant experiments, Ratych *et al.* [35] proposed that the entire xanthine oxidase-based free radical-generating system is operative within the endothelial cell itself. In some organs this endothelial cell injury may also act as an initial trigger to attract and activate neutrophils which may actually cause most of the damage.

Intermediates in enzymic and peroxidative action

Free radicals are also involved in the mechanism of action of certain enzymes, for example, the iron–sulphur enzyme ribonucleoside diphosphate reductase, or the haem enzymes cytochrome P-450 and prostaglandin synthase. Arachidonic acid in stimulated cells may be mobilized by activation of either phospholipase A_2 acting on phosphatidylethanolamine, phosphatidylcholine of plasmalogens, or phospholipase C and diacylglycerol lipase acting sequentially on phosphatidylinositol derivatives, to initiate prostaglandin and leukotriene synthesis. The enzymic oxidation of arachidonic acid during eicosanoid biosynthesis is accompanied by the generation of hydroperoxides and formation of oxygen radicals. The actions of prostaglandin synthase and lipoxygenase operate through mechanisms involving free radical intermediates. The conversion of the hydroperoxide prostaglandin G_2 (PGG$_2$) to prostaglandin H_2 (PGH$_2$) [36] during prostaglandin synthesis yields reactive oxygen species, an active haem iron–oxygen ferryl species being formed during the peroxidase reaction [37]. It has also been proposed that the haem iron in the enzyme must be reduced for maximal activity [38], which can be effected by superoxide radical, lipid hydroperoxides and hydrogen peroxide.

Once arachidonate is released, it can interact with prostaglandin endoperoxide synthase (PGH synthase), which exhibits both cyclo-oxygenase or bisoxygenation activity and peroxidative activity, or with lipoxygenases in a controlled and stereospecific manner to yield initially peroxides, namely PGG$_2$ and hydroperoxyeicosatetraenoic acid. The initial products of prostaglandin

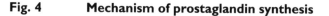

Fig. 4   **Mechanism of prostaglandin synthesis**

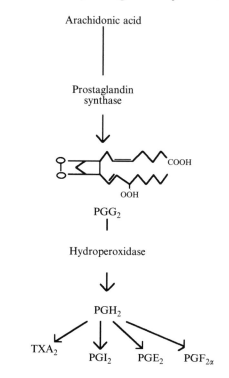

Abbreviations used: PG, prostaglandin; TX, thromboxane.

and leukotriene synthesis are peroxides. The sequence of reactions is illustrated in Fig. 4 and Fig. 5.

The peroxidase activity of PGH synthase (reviewed in [39]) catalyses the reduction of fatty acid hydroperoxides, including PGG_2, to alcohols, including PGH_2, with the two reducing equivalents supplied by a reducing co-substrate (Fig. 6). The alcohol is produced by a direct simultaneous two-electron reduction of the hydroperoxide, typical of the action of classical haem peroxidases [40]. The peroxidase is less active towards hydrogen peroxide [41].

A characteristic feature of the haem peroxidases, the haem prosthetic group being essential for such peroxidative activity, is the formation of spectroscopically detectable radical intermediates during the catalytic cycle. The nature of the e.p.r. signal suggests that the free radical intermediate is a tyrosyl radical [42]. For catalytic turnover of prostaglandin synthase peroxidase to

Fig. 5   **Mechanism of lipoxygenase action**

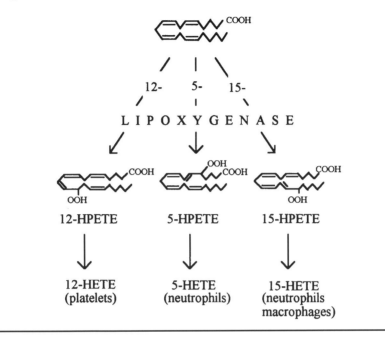

12-HPETE   5-HPETE   15-HPETE

12-HETE   5-HETE   15-HETE
(platelets)   (neutrophils)   (neutrophils
                                    macrophages)

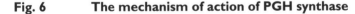

Fig. 6   **The mechanism of action of PGH synthase**

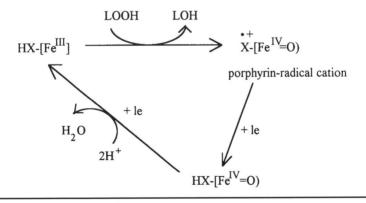

occur, the higher oxidation states of the enzyme must be reduced. A variety of compounds support the hydroperoxide reduction, electron-rich molecules being the preferred physiological reductants. Physiologically, such compounds might be urate [43–45] (plasma mean concentration, 400 μM) and glutathione, relatively poorly reducing but present in cells at very high concentrations (2–5 μM). Lipoxygenases catalyse the regio-specific and stereo-selective oxygenation of unsaturated fatty acids. The mammalian enzymes have been detected in human platelets, lung, kidney, testes and white blood cells. The leukotrienes, derived from enzymic activity on arachidonic acid, have effects on neutrophil migration and aggregation, release of lysosomal enzymes, capillary permeability, induction of pain and smooth muscle contraction [46].

Endothelial-derived relaxing factor

NO is synthesized in a variety of cells and tissues through an L-arginine-dependent NO synthase (see Chapter 4). NO from endothelial cells, otherwise known as endothelial-derived relaxing factor [47], is involved in the regulation of vascular tone, inducing the relaxation of smooth muscle cells through the activation of the haem enzyme guanylate cyclase. Macrophage-derived NO has been implicated in the killing of tumour cells and bacteria [48].

It has been shown that NO inhibits the respiratory burst enzyme responsible for generating superoxide radical in activated neutrophils, which points to the unlikelihood of both NO and $O_2^{-\cdot}$ being produced concomitantly in neutrophils [49]. This is a highly significant observation since the product of their interaction (rate constant $6.7 \times 10^9 \, \text{mol}^{-1} \, \text{s}^{-1}$) is peroxynitrite (eqn. 8), a potent oxidant capable of initiating lipid peroxidation, oxidizing sulphydryl groups on proteins, inducing the nitration of tyrosine residues and oxidizing α-tocopherol in LDLs [2,50–52].

$$O_2^{-\cdot} + NO^{\cdot} \rightarrow ONOO^- \tag{8}$$

where $ONOO^-$ is the peroxynitrite anion. This reaction eventually produces nitrites and nitrates. The biochemical, physiological and pathological aspects of NO are discussed in Chapter 4 by Darley-Usmar and co-workers.

Antioxidants and their action

The definition of an antioxidant that is currently most acceptable is any substance which, when present at low concentrations compared with those of the oxidizable substrate, significantly delays or inhibits oxidation of that substrate. The body is equipped with a range of antioxidants to protect against excessive radical generation and the consequences thereof [53]. Those found intracellularly are appropriately located for scavenging aberrant free radical species. Extracellular antioxidants have the role of intercepting propagating radical reactions and removing delocalized metal ions and decompartmentalized haem proteins, by sequestering them in forms incapable of stimulating free-radical reactions.

Antioxidant enzymes

The antioxidant enzymes involved in removing reactive oxygen species are the superoxide dismutases [54], catalase [55], glutathione peroxidase [56] and other peroxidases. Other essential enzymes which are involved in an anti-oxidant capacity are those promoting the synthesis of such antioxidant com-pounds as glutathione, ascorbate, urate, bilirubin and ubiquinol, and those preventing the formation of reactive oxygen species, e.g. glutathione trans-ferases and DT-diaphorase, and those promoting the regeneration of anti-oxidant compounds, namely glutathione reductase and semiquinone reductases.

Plasma antioxidants

The major plasma antioxidants include ascorbate, albumin, urate, bilirubin, the iron-handling systems caeruloplasmin and transferrin, the haem-removing antioxidants haptoglobin and haemopexin, and tocopherols and carotenoids, which are lipoprotein-soluble antioxidants.

Ascorbate

This water-soluble antioxidant is also found in specific intracellular locations, particularly muscle, the adrenals and the eye. The most important chemical property of ascorbate is its ease of oxidation either by one- or two-electron transfer. Both the 2- and 3-hydroxyl groups must be unsubstituted for anti-oxidant activity [57]. During its antioxidant action, ascorbic acid undergoes a two-electron oxidation to dehydroascorbate with intermediate formation of the ascorbyl radical [58]. Dehydroascorbate is relatively unstable and can be reduced back to ascorbate or hydrolysed to diketogulonic acid. It reacts with oxygen and hydrogen peroxide, and scavenges oxygen radicals (superoxide, hydroperoxyl and hydroxyl radical) and singlet oxygen [59–61]. In the pres-ence of transition metals, especially iron(III) or copper(II) ions, the autoxida-tion of ascorbate is catalysed, forming dehydroascorbate with the production of hydrogen peroxide [62]. The ascorbate monoanion is involved in an inter-mediate complex.

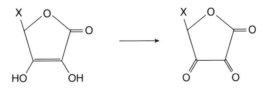

where $X = CH_2(OH)CH(OH)^{-\cdot}$

Thus a number of metal-chelating agents will retard the autoxidation of ascorbate, including EDTA, citrate, oxalate, histidine, urate and flavonoids. This is particularly important when considering the antioxidant properties of foods [63].

Albumin

Albumin, the major protein of human plasma, binds to copper and iron, the latter weakly. The sulphydryl group of albumin may also be important at specific locations in intercepting hypochlorite.

Urate

Urate is traditionally seen as a metabolically inert end-product of purine metabolism in man, in an NAD-dependent reaction of xanthine dehydrogenase or oxygen-dependent reaction of xanthine oxidase. It has been proven to be a selective antioxidant (reviewed in [64]) capable of chelation of catalytically active iron [65]; reaction with hypochlorous acid [66]; and attenuation of the ozone-induced oxidation of lipids, lipoproteins and unsaturated fatty acids [67–69]. Currently, the tendency still remains to regard urate as a risk factor for atherosclerosis and coronary heart disease [70–72], although recent epidemiological studies have not confirmed the predicted associations. Several studies have suggested that the urate radical may be a reactive oxidant and, therefore, its maximal effectiveness as an antioxidant might be in the presence of a potential regenerating agent such as ascorbate [73], although urate has also been described as a protective antioxidant for ascorbate [74]. It is, however, unlikely that this would be physiologically relevant since plasma ascorbate seems to be utilized before urate [75].

Bilirubin

Bilirubin is able to scavenge singlet oxygen and peroxyl radicals [76]. It has been proposed that bilirubin bound to human albumin contributes significantly to the non-enzymic antioxidant defences in human plasma.

α-Tocopherol

α-Tocopherol is the major lipid-soluble, chain-breaking antioxidant in plasma and in cell membranes [77]. It inhibits amplification of peroxidation by intercepting propagating lipid chains, by reducing peroxyl radicals to hydroperoxides. α-Tocopherol reacts with peroxyl radicals with a rate constant of approximately 10^6 mol^{-1} s^{-1} [78]. However, in the presence of haem proteins or iron or copper complexes, lipid peroxides can continue cycling to peroxyl radicals which can be intercepted by tocopherol; reductive decomposition of peroxides to alkoxyl radicals and interaction with α-tocopherol forms hydroxyl derivatives which terminate the sequence.

It has been proposed that the α-tocopheroxyl radical can be recycled back to tocopherol by ascorbate, producing the ascorbyl radical [79,80]. The location of α-tocopherol with its phytyl tail in the membrane parallel to the fatty acyl chains of the phospholipids, and its phenolic hydroxyl group at the membrane–water interface near the polar head-groups of the phospholipid bilayer, enables ascorbate to donate hydrogen atoms to the tocopheroxyl radical. The suitability of ascorbate and tocopherol as chain-breaking antioxidants is exemplified [81,82] by the fact that they are effective in relatively small amounts and their radical states are relatively unreactive, in either reducing or oxidizing capacities. Recent studies in experimental chemical systems have described systems in which the α-tocopheroxyl radical can act as a pro-oxidant [83]. This is perhaps not so surprising, in view of the well-known characteristic of many antioxidants in their assumption of the characteristics of pro-oxidants at high concentration.

Carotenoids
A number of polyenes and carotenoids found in animal tissue are associated with lipid antioxidant functions [84]. In addition, in humans, β-carotene, α-carotene and cryptoxanthine are converted to vitamin A, whereas lutein and lycopene are not [85]. The antioxidant function of carotene is attributed to its molecular structure which allows the quenching of singlet oxygen and scavenging of free radicals. β-Carotene may exert its antioxidant function through its ability to interact with a radical, yielding a less-reactive, resonance-stabilized, carbon-centred radical species [86], whereby the chain-carrying peroxyl radicals add covalently to the conjugated system of β-carotene. β-Carotene appears to exert its optimal effectiveness at low oxygen tensions. It has been proposed that lycopene is the most efficient singlet oxygen quencher [87].

Ubiquinol
Ubiquinol [88] has recently been proposed to be a chain-breaking antioxidant [89], in LDLs as the first line of defence [90], and in liposomal systems [91].

Haptoglobin
Haptoglobin binds free haemoglobin released from erythrocytes, preventing iron from being made available and the haem protein from propagating lipid peroxidation.

Haemopexin
Haemopexin binds free haem, thus inhibiting haem-induced propagation of lipid peroxidation.

Caeruloplasmin
The copper-containing ferroxidase catalyses iron(II) conversion to iron(III) [92], enabling its subsequent removal by binding to transferrin.

Transferrin
Transferrin is a protein which binds ferric iron (2 mole per mole of protein) with a binding constant of 10^{20}, making it unavailable for catalysing radical reactions. This iron-transporting protein of the blood delivers it to the storage

sites on ferritin in cells. The iron-binding sites on transferrin are normally only 30% occupied, explaining the lack of free or available iron in human plasma.

The hierarchy of antioxidant effectiveness in plasma has been defined from studies *in vitro* [93] as

Ascorbate = protein thiols > bilirubin > urate > tocopherol

against radicals generated in the aqueous phase, such that plasma depleted of ascorbate but replete in the rest is vulnerable to oxidative stress and susceptible to lipid oxidation from radicals generated in the aqueous phase. However, plasma replete in ascorbate but deficient in the others is resistant to such oxidation until the ascorbate is consumed. The lipophilic antioxidants of plasma are located mainly in the lipoproteins. In the LDL fraction, the polyunsaturated fatty acids of the phospholipids constituting the outer monolayer are protected by α-tocopherol, with approximately 10 mole per mole of fatty acid, whereas the inner core of cholesteryl esters contains the carotenoids — β-carotene, lycopene, lutein, phytofluene, zeaxanthin and α-carotene — which have had the role of protection of the polyunsaturated fatty acid chains against oxidation assigned to them. The normal ranges of antioxidants in plasma and LDL are listed in Table 1 and Table 2.

Table 1   Normal range of concentrations of adult human plasma antioxidants

Antioxidant	Plasma concentration
Albumin	50 g/l
Urate	180–420 μM
Ascorbate	34–111 μM
α-Tocopherol	14–44 μM
Bilirubin	<20 μM
Reduced glutathione	1–4 μM
Iron-handling proteins	
Transferrin	1.8–3.3 g/l
Caeruloplasmin	0.18–0.4 g/l
Haptoglobin	0.5–3.6 g/l
Haemopexin	0.6–1.0 g/l

Data taken from [94–96].

Table 2   Ranges of values for lipophilic antioxidant levels in LDL (mol of antioxidant/mol of LDL)

Lipophilic antioxidant	Level in LDL (mol/mol of LDL)
β-Carotene	0.03–1.87
Lycopene	0.03–0.7
Lutein + zeaxanthin	0.01–0.16
α-Carotene	0.02–0.52
Ubiquinol 10	0.03–0.35
Phytofluene	0.02–0.11
Cantaxanthin	0.01–0.24
α-Tocopherol	2.90–15.74
γ-Tocopherol	0.07–1.70

Data taken from [97].

Recent studies have pointed to the importance of the antioxidant nutrients vitamin C, vitamin E and β-carotene in maintaining health, in contributing to a decreased incidence of disease and in protecting against the recurrence of pathological events. The WHO cross-cultural epidemiological survey [98] of 16 European countries showed an inverse correlation between vitamin E levels in the blood and the incidence of mortality from ischaemic heart disease. The Harvard Male Physicians' Study, supplementing with 50 mg β-carotene on alternate days, showed a 44% reduction in all major coronary events [99]. The time is approaching when it is becoming possible to define the intake of antioxidant nutrients that is associated with a low subsequent incidence of coronary heart disease. The recent Health Professionals Study [100,101], on groups of 40000 males and 87000 females, showed a 37% reduction in risk for males from coronary heart disease after daily supplementation with 100 IU of vitamin E for at least 2 years and a 41% reduction in risk for females with 200 IU over the same minimum period.

A major question in considering the mechanisms relating antioxidant status in the blood with decreased risk of coronary heart disease is the relationship between plasma antioxidant levels and the total antioxidant activity, which might depend on synergistic interactions between antioxidants. Many studies *in vitro* have discussed the synergistic interactions between vitamin E and vitamin C, and of vitamin E with β-carotene. As early as 1941, Golumbic and Mattill [102] showed that the combined antioxidant effects of vitamin C and vitamin E in protecting fats against oxidation were greater than the sum of their individual contributions, and that the former was protecting the latter from oxidation. Subsequently, others have confirmed the synergistic action *in vitro* and shown that the water-soluble vitamin C acts to keep vitamin E, located in a lipophilic region, in its reduced state [77,79,80,103–104].

In addition, based on the standard one-electron reduction potentials, Buettner [81] has predicted a hierarchy of antioxidants, from highly oxidizing to highly reducing species, in terms of the ability of each reducing species to donate an electron (or hydrogen atom) to any oxidized species listed above. Thus, in general, in a cascade of free radical reactions, each reaction in the sequence will generate less-reactive radicals, with antioxidants producing the least reactive radicals of all. However, in the presence of transition metals, such as iron or copper, and oxygen, this would not be the case, but rather the reactivity would be amplified. These potentials are also in agreement with the experimental data suggesting the ability of α-tocopherol and ascorbate to co-operate in the protection of lipid against peroxidation [102,105,106], although this has not been shown *in vivo*.

Factors controlling the release of free radicals in disease states

Oxidative stress may derive from excess endogenous oxygen radical generation accompanying pathological states or may be due to exogenous sources of free radicals, such as irradiation, hyperoxia, drugs or toxins (Fig. 7). Reactive free radical species may oxidatively damage the polyunsaturated fatty acids of

Fig. 7   Tissue damage arising from exogenous sources of free radicals or accompanying disease states due to endogenous factors

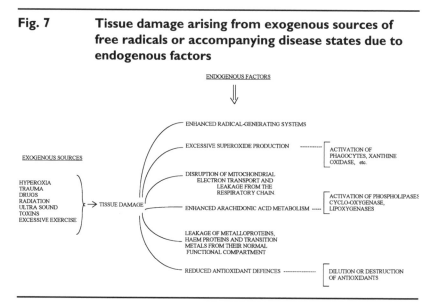

membrane lipids (reviewed in [107]) or lipoproteins, oxidize cholesterol, modify the structural and functional integrity of proteins, oxidize carbohydrates or induce scissions in the base of carbohydrate components of nucleic acids.

Peroxidation of polyunsaturated fatty acid side-chains

Polyunsaturated fatty acids are highly susceptible to free radical attack. Thus, lipid peroxidation may be initiated by any primary free radical with sufficient reactivity to subtract an allylic hydrogen atom (Fig. 8) from a reactive methylene group of polyunsaturated fatty acid side-chains. The formation of the dienyl radical is followed by bond rearrangement that results in stabilization by conjugated diene formation, and, after oxygen uptake, the formation of the

Fig. 8   The mechanism of lipid peroxidation

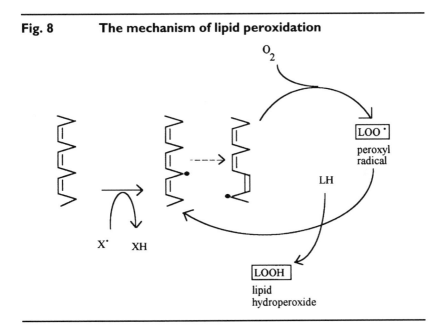

peroxyl radical. Propagation reactions follow, leading to the formation of lipid hydroperoxides. This propagation phase can be repeated many times as indicated. Thus, an initial event triggering lipid peroxidation can be amplified, as long as oxygen supplies and unoxidized polyunsaturated fatty acid chains are available.

The accumulation of hydroperoxides and their subsequent decomposition to alkoxyl and peroxyl radicals can accelerate the chain reaction of polyunsaturated fatty acid peroxidation, leading to oxidative damage to cells, membranes and lipoproteins. It is well-recognized that haem proteins, through their redox cycling properties, may play a role in promoting oxidative stress by catalysing the decomposition of hydroperoxides [108–110], generating alkoxyl (LO˙) and peroxyl (LOO˙) radical species (see eqns. 7–9) which can exacerbate the peroxidative process, initiating further rounds of lipid peroxidation as well as recycling the haem proteins for further oxidative events.

$$LOOH + HX\text{-}Fe^{II} \longrightarrow LO^{\cdot} + HX\text{-}Fe^{III} + OH^{-} \tag{9}$$

$$LOOH + HX\text{-}Fe^{III} \longrightarrow LOO^{\cdot} + HX\text{-}Fe^{II} + H^{+} \tag{10}$$

$$\longrightarrow LO^{\cdot} + HX(Fe^{IV}\!\!=\!\!O) + H^{+} \tag{11}$$

$$LO^{\cdot} + LH \longrightarrow LOH + L^{\cdot} \tag{12}$$

$$L^{\cdot} + O_2 \longrightarrow LOO^{\cdot} \tag{13}$$

$$LOO^{\cdot} + LH \longrightarrow LOOH + L^{\cdot} \tag{14}$$

The lipid peroxyl radicals, formed during the modification of the polyunsaturated fatty acid side-chains of lipids, can amplify lipid peroxidation, oxidize cholesterol and react with proteins, impairing the functions of critical enzyme and receptor systems.

The potential consequences of the peroxidation of membrane lipids include loss of polyunsaturated fatty acids, decreased lipid fluidity, altered membrane permeability, effects on membrane-associated enzymes, altered ion transport, release of material from subcellular compartments and the generation of cytotoxic metabolites of lipid hydroperoxides. The major lipid peroxidation products of physiological significance are lipid peroxides (LOOH), epoxy fatty acids and 4-hydroxyalkenals. Lipid peroxides stimulate prostaglandin synthesis by activating cyclo-oxygenase, control cell proliferation and affect cell growth, modulate the activity of phospholipases and show second messenger effects through the reduction of thiol groups to essential disulphides [111]. Epoxy fatty acids affect hormone secretion, and 4-hydroxyalkenals affect adenylate cyclase and phospholipase C activities, reduce cell growth and promote cell differentiation, inhibit platelet aggregation, block macrophage action and block thiol groups.

Cleavage of the carbon bonds during lipid peroxidation reactions results in the formation of aldehyde products, such as cytotoxic alkanals and alkenals, as well as alkanes. The breakdown products of lipid peroxidation, alkanals such as malonaldehyde [112] and alkenals and hydroxyalkenals such as 4-hydroxynonenal [113] are toxic, undergoing Schiff-base formation with amino groups, interacting with thiol groups, inactivating enzymes and demonstrating cytotoxic properties. 4-Hydroxynonenal inhibits platelet aggregation, modifies adenylate cyclase activity and is a substrate for the glutathione transferases.

Oxidant damage to proteins

Radical generation at inappropriate sites may lead to protein destruction since they are also critical targets for free radical attack, both intracellularly and

Fig. 9   Oxidation products of protein constituents mediated by free radicals

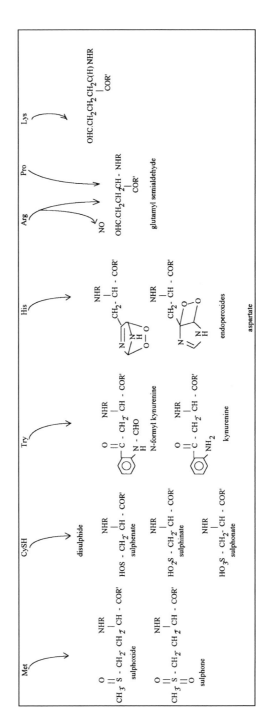

extracellularly. Proteins may be directly damaged through specific interactions of oxidants or free radicals with particularly susceptible amino acids. Several amino acyl constituents crucial for protein function are particularly vulnerable to radical damage (Fig. 9) [114–116].

Protein damage by free radical species such as peroxyl radicals and hydroxyl radicals, or active oxygen species such as hypochlorite and hydrogen peroxide, may occur through a variety of mechanisms including amino acid oxidation, deamination, decarboxylation, ring scission and cross-linking. In addition, protein hydroperoxides have been described as novel reactive products of radical attack on proteins, shown *in vitro* [117]. Some amino acid residues are more susceptible than others to oxidant attack, and exposure of proteins to free radical-generating systems may induce tertiary structural changes as a consequence of modifications to specific amino acid side-chains. As secondary structure is stabilized by hydrogen bonding between peptide groups, interactions of radical species with the polypeptide backbone and interference with the functional groups of the peptide bonds may cause secondary structural modifications and protein unfolding (reviewed in [118]).

It has been proposed that in some instances, when protein radicals are formed at a specific amino acyl site, they can be rapidly transferred to other sites within the protein infrastructure [119] from:

$$\text{methionine} \rightarrow \text{tryptophan} \rightarrow \text{tyrosine} \rightarrow \text{cysteine}$$

Hypochlorous acid, in particular, attacks targets at the site of its production, especially with such amino acyl protein constituents as amino groups, sulphydryl groups, and methionine and tyrosine residues [120,121]. It has been suggested that inactivation of α_1-antiproteinase *in vivo* is due to hypochlorite-mediated oxidation of an essential methionine residue at the active site of the enzyme [122]. Inactivation of the α_1-proteinase inhibitor may allow proteases to be active, causing emphysema.

Proteins are also particularly susceptible to attack from free radical intermediates of lipid peroxidation, such as alkoxyl and peroxyl radicals. These may react with amino acids, such as histidine and proline, in proteins closely associated with peroxidizing lipids. The consequences of such damage may be impaired enzymic activity and modified membrane and cellular function, resulting from aggregation or cross-linking of receptor proteins for example, or protein degradation and fragmentation, depending on the nature of the vulnerable protein component and the attacking radical species [123,124]. Damage to the ion transport proteins of the membrane, the Na^+-, K^+- and Ca^{2+}-ATPases with vulnerable reduced thiol groups at their active centres, might affect ionic homoeostasis, leading to calcium accumulation, for example. Consequently, the potential for calcium-mediated activation of phospho-

Fig. 10 Mechanisms of glucose oxidation

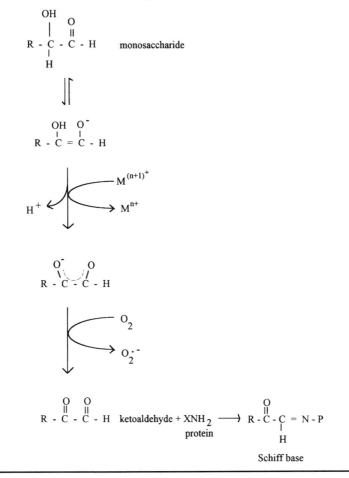

lipases, proteases, or the accumulation of mitochondrial calcium may lead to extensive membrane damage and cellular deterioration.

Carbonyl derivatives as decomposition products of lipid peroxidation or monosaccharide oxidation (see below) can interact with amino groups on protein amino acyl side-chains, thus altering their charge and nature. The former mechanism has been proposed as a contributing factor in the sequence of events in the oxidative modification of LDLs, facilitating recognition by scavenger receptors on macrophages (see Chapter 5); the binding of complex mixtures of aldehydes including malonaldehyde and 4-hydroxynonenal, secondary metabolites of the peroxidation of polyunsaturated fatty acyl chains, to lysine residues on the apo B protein portion of LDLs decreases the positive charge on the surface of the LDL and limits its uptake by the conventional

Fig. 11   The Maillard reaction

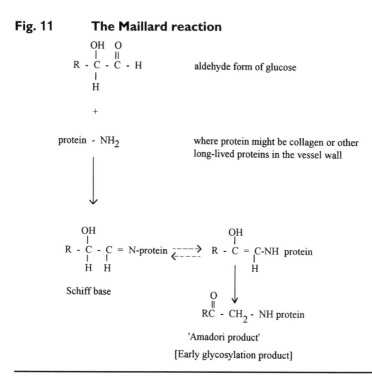

OH O
| ||
R - C - C - H   aldehyde form of glucose
    |
    H

+

protein - NH₂   where protein might be collagen or other
                         long-lived proteins in the vessel wall

      OH   OH
      | |
R - C - C = N-protein ----→   R - C = C-NH protein
      | | ←---- | |
      H   H   H

Schiff base   O
                                     ||
                             RC - CH₂ - NH protein

                         'Amadori product'
                      [Early glycosylation product]

LDL receptor on cells [125–127]. Instead, it becomes recognizable by the scavenger receptors on macrophages, forming cholesterol-laden foam cells which contribute towards fatty streak formation in atherosclerosis.

Carbohydrate oxidation and consequences for protein function

Two alternative mechanisms by which glucose may induce structural changes in proteins have recently become prominent [128–130]. Monosaccharides are oxidized when catalysed by trace amounts of transition metals, generating free radicals, hydrogen peroxide and reactive dicarbonyls directly [131,132]. The process of glucose oxidation, in a transition-metal-dependent reaction, can lead to protein damage by free radicals and by covalent binding of the carbonyl products to protein components (Fig. 10). The Maillard reaction describes the non-enzymic glycation of proteins (Fig. 11). Glucose is considered to be toxic because of its ability to behave chemically as an aldehyde and is known to form chemically reversible early glycosylation products with protein (Schiff bases) at a rate proportional to the glucose concentration. These Schiff bases then rearrange to form the more stable Amadori-type early glycosylation products [133]. Protein which has been glycated *in vitro* is conformationally altered. The amount of early glycosylation products *in vivo* in diabetics, whether on haemoglobin or basement membrane, increases when blood glucose levels are high and returns to normal after the glucose levels are normalized by treatment.

The subsequent degradation or glycoxidation of protein-bound Amadori products in a transition metal-dependent process can yield further oxidants and protein-reactive aldehydes [128]. Thus, some of the early glycosylation products on collagen and other long-lived proteins of the vessel wall undergo a slow, complex series of chemical rearrangements to form irreversible advanced glycosylation end-products. A number of these irreversible end-products are capable of forming covalent bonds with amino groups on other proteins, forming cross-links. It has been proposed that hyperglycaemia in diabetes may involve covalent cross-linking of extravasated plasma lipoproteins to matrix lipoproteins by advanced glycosylation end-products, retarding the rate of cholesterol efflux and accelerating the development of vascular disease.

A number of studies *in vitro* have shown that the production of protein-reactive dicarbonyl compounds [130], hydrogen peroxide [134] and oxidants [128] by glucose in solution (glucose autoxidation) is inhibited in the presence of albumin. This protein is reasonably ubiquitous, perhaps suggesting that oxidant production by glucose autoxidation *in vivo* is, if it occurs, a localized event. Essentially, oxidative damage of proteins by glucose autoxidation has been shown *in vitro* to be decreased by increasing concentrations of albumin in an apparently exponential manner [132]. In the circulation and the extracellular fluid of some tissues, such as the arterial wall at sites of haemodynamic injury, protein concentrations are unlikely to be consistent with glucose autoxidation. Further evidence cited against the significance of glucose autoxidation includes studies suggesting that the chemistries of glucose autoxidation and glycoxidation compete for the open-chain form of glucose necessary for enediol and Schiff-base formation, respectively. There is also some suggestion that glycation occurs at a more significant rate than glucose autoxidation [135].

Interestingly, some Maillard reaction products have antioxidant activity [136]; the Maillard reaction products from the amino acid–sugar combination of histidine and glucose have stronger antioxidant properties than other combinations [137].

Is there a role for iron or haem proteins in the amplification of lipid peroxidation in atherosclerosis?

Evidence is accumulating from studies *in vitro* that LDL can be oxidatively modified by: (i) cells in culture, including endothelial cells [138], arterial smooth muscle cells [139] and macrophages [140–142]; (ii) ruptured erythrocytes [143] and myocytes [144]; (iii) co-incubation with transition metal ions, such as copper [97], or with haem proteins such as haemoglobin and myoglobin [140,145]. LDL is subsequently recognized and rapidly taken up by scavenger receptors on target macrophages. The extensive studies of Esterbauer *et al.* [97] have shown that the endogenous antioxidant status of LDL is one of the major determinants of its oxidizability. In addition, the lag phase to oxidation of LDL is reflected in the amount of peroxides present before the oxidative challenge [146] as well as being attributed to the antioxidant status of the LDL [97] (see Chapter 3); (iv) 15-lipoxygenase in macrophages [147].

The mechanism by which LDL becomes oxidized *in vivo* is not clear. It is not known whether a specific initiating radical species is essential or whether the propagation of peroxidation, subsequent to lipoxygenase-mediated hydroperoxide formation, is the major likely priming event. If the former, what is the probable initiating agent, where is it located and what activates it? If the latter, are the lipoxygenases involved or are hydroperoxides incorporated from the diet; in these cases what might be the mediator of the propagation of the oxidation event?

Cell-induced modification of LDL in culture *in vitro* has been demonstrated to be mediated by free radicals. All the cell types have been shown to release superoxide radicals, albeit by different mechanisms and at different rates. Thus, addition of SOD has an inhibitory effect on the oxidative modification, although the response varies according to cell type, implicating superoxide radical in the mechanism of cell-mediated modification [148,149]. Neither catalase nor mannitol inhibit LDL oxidation by smooth muscle cells, thus a Fenton-driven mechanism can be discounted [149] if smooth muscle cell-mediated oxidation is deemed to be an important contributor to the oxidative process. The significance of superoxide radical in the initiation, but not in the propagation, of LDL oxidation in cultures of monocytes/macrophages is indicated by experiments showing inhibition of the oxidative modification by SOD only if the antioxidant is added within a few hours of the initiation of the incubation. However, an antioxidant such as butylated hydroxytoluene, a lipid-chain-breaking antioxidant as well as a hydroxyl radical scavenger, is effective in inhibiting the oxidative modification as late as 11 h after the onset of incubation. It is important to note that small amounts of iron in the medium are an absolute requirement for oxidation of LDL by cultured macrophages [142].

If the superoxide released from these cells is a mediator of the oxidative modification of LDL in the artery wall, what amplifies its reactivity to enable initiation of peroxidation? Are delocalized haem proteins from ruptured erythrocytes or myocytes, or decompartmentalized iron or copper, involved? Our recent studies have shown that haem proteins and those released from ruptured myocytes and erythrocytes are capable of mediating the oxidative modification of LDL *in vitro* and that this interaction is peroxide-dependent [143,144]. Another possibility is that peroxynitrite plays a key role *in vivo* (see Chapter 4 by Darley-Usmar *et al.*). There is still much work to be carried out to resolve these issues and to understand the relevant mechanisms *in vivo*.

Several studies have questioned whether oxidized LDL can be detected in the circulation of patients with coronary heart disease. Studies from Sweden [150] have associated the susceptibility of LDL to oxidation with the severity of coronary atherosclerosis, and studies from Canada [151] have demonstrated that LDL from middle-aged men with coronary heart disease contains oxidized cholesterol.

Our recent studies have monitored the susceptibility to oxidation of LDLs from the blood of patients with carotid or femoral artery atherosclerosis and related this susceptibility to the progression of the disease [152]. LDLs were isolated from the blood of 37 patients (35 male, 2 female) with a demonstrable atherosclerotic plaque detected by duplex scanning. The susceptibility to oxidation of the LDL induced by an exogenous oxidative stress (5 μM metmyoglobin) was assessed by three methods: (i) measuring the breakdown products of lipid peroxidation; (ii) by observing spectroscopically the increased formation of conjugated dienes; and (iii) monitoring the change in the surface charge of the apolipoprotein portion of the LDL.

The progression of the atherosclerotic plaque was assessed by measuring the maximum velocity of blood through the narrowest portion of the vessel at inclusion and after 1 year. Of the 37 samples taken, 29 were found to have LDLs that were partially oxidized, whereas 8 samples showed LDLs whose state of oxidation was within the normal range. Progression of the atheromatous plaque occurred in 19 of the 29 patients whose lipoproteins were partially oxidized compared with only 2 of the 8 patients with normal lipoproteins ($p = 0.05$, Fisher's exact test).

These data support an association between the progression of atherosclerotic plaques in carotid and femoral vessels and the susceptibility to oxidation of LDLs.

Sources of free radicals in reperfusion injury

Reperfusion injury (see Chapter 8; reviewed in [153–155]) can be defined as the damage that occurs to an organ during the resumption of blood flow, after an episode of ischaemia. This is quite separate from the injury caused by ischaemia *per se*.

When tissues are deprived of oxygen they are injured and, after a period, the injury becomes irreversible. The duration of this period depends on the extent of oxygen deprivation (hypoxia or ischaemia) and the tissue in question. There are several clinical settings in which the myocardium is exposed to transient ischaemia, including unstable angina, evolving myocardial infarction and certain therapeutic procedures, such as percutaneous transluminal angioplasty, thrombolysis and cardiopulmonary bypass during cardiac surgery [155]. Prolonged ischaemia, such as that occurring after myocardial infarction or during long-term coronary bypass procedures, can cause serious damage to the myocardium. Paradoxically, while reperfusion of the ischaemic myocardium is necessary for the restoration of normal metabolic activity, the return of normotensive oxygen to the myocardium can be detrimental, leading to suboptimal myocardial salvage. The phenomenon whereby necrosis of previously viable myocardium is attributed to reperfusion rather than to the preceding ischaemic event is referred to as 'reperfusion or reoxygenation injury'. Clinical manifestations of the underlying pathological events of reperfusion injury may include both electrical and contractile dysfunction of the myocardium, leading to arrhythmias and ultimately to mechanical failure of the heart.

The evolution of the reperfusion-associated contractile and rhythmic disturbances appears to involve a variety of events, including (i) a rapid influx of calcium into the myocardial cells, possibly as a result of membrane defects or sodium–calcium exchange [156]; (ii) reduced reperfusion of the previously ischaemic area by endothelial cell swelling, interstitial oedema or neutrophil plugging, prolonging ischaemia, and (iii) activation of neutrophils, leading to the release of a variety of cytotoxic agents including proteolytic enzymes from inflammatory cells at the site of injury. More myocardial damage and, ultimately, lysis of the myocytes may occur, leading to the presence of creatine kinase, lactate dehydrogenase and myoglobin in the plasma [10]. Elevated free radical formation on reperfusion has been proposed to be a significant factor in all these mechanisms and this occurs in the early seconds after reperfusion [157,158]. In fact, it has been argued that the ischaemic myocardium is more susceptible to free radical damage on reperfusion, since the endogenous protective antioxidant mechanisms are diminished during ischaemia [159–161].

A wide variety of cells, organelles and enzymes may be potential sources of free radicals during myocardial post-ischaemic reperfusion injury, and are interrelated in a complex fashion. This includes adhesion and activation of leucocytes at a site of injury on the endothelium after ischaemic insult, aberrantly functioning mitochondria and the xanthine oxidase system of the vascular endothelial cells. Oxygen-derived free radicals are produced by activated leucocytes, neutrophils, and so on (reviewed in [155]), which infiltrate the ischaemic and reperfused myocardium as a normal component of the acute inflammatory response and attack viable myocytes primarily through the release of free radicals. As an important part of their antimicrobial mechanisms, the neutrophil generates superoxide and other reactive species of oxygen through a membrane-bound NADPH oxidase (as described earlier), activated by a variety of stimuli including components of the complement system, C3a for example. It has been proposed that the ischaemic myocardial tissue gives rise to a tissue protease that activates complement and induces migration of neutrophils into the primed myocardium. Other chemoattractants, including leukotriene B_4, are also generated in response to myocardial tissue injury. This allows for rapid access of the inflammatory cells to the primed myocardial region at risk. Superoxide radical produced by the NADPH oxidase of activated phagocytes initiates a cascade of events leading to the formation of hydrogen peroxide, hypochlorous acid and monochloramines, which normally function within the phagocytic vacuole to provide a defence mechanism against micro-organisms. Reactive oxygen species have deleterious effects on surrounding cells and tissues when they are released into the extracellular environment. Released superoxide amplifies the inflammatory response by activation of a latent chemoattractant present in extracellular fluids. Leucocyte depletion has been noted to decrease damage due to ischaemia and reperfusion, as measured by reduced infarct size, to a degree comparable to the reduction seen on applying scavengers of superoxide radical and hydrogen peroxide. There is no doubt that leucocytes concentrate in the ischaemic myocardium. The question is: are leucocytes attacking viable cells in the reperfused tissue and are they in place early enough to account for injury incurred at the time of reperfusion [155]?

A further potential source of oxygen-derived free radicals in reperfusion injury is the enzyme xanthine oxidase (reviewed in [162,32]), an enzyme associated with the vascular endothelial cells. It may play an important role in the brain, but its presence in the myocytes of the human heart is debated. Decreased energy stores during ischaemia result in the accumulation of adenine nucleotides. During reperfusion, metabolism of adenine nucleotides via the xanthine oxidase pathway is a probable source of oxygen radicals in the brain. Xanthine dehydrogenase may be converted to xanthine oxidase, on oxidation of sulphydryl groups, or on activation of a calcium-dependent protease by increased cytosolic calcium levels made available from a breakdown of homoeostatic mechanisms occurring during hypoxia/ischaemia. Xanthine oxidase catalyses the conversion of accumulated purine metabolites, such as hypoxanthine, to urate on reperfusion and generates superoxide radical and hydrogen peroxide. In organs other than the heart, the endothelial trigger mechanism based on xanthine oxidase is given a predominant role in superoxide generation in reperfusion injury.

Intracellularly, radicals may also arise by electron leakage from the mitochondrial electron transport chain [163] as a consequence of the accumulation of reducing equivalents during the ischaemic period, when oxygen is not available to act as the terminal electron acceptor of the respiratory chain.

The myocardium contains abundant SOD and the superoxide formed upon return of molecular oxygen to the myocardium will therefore be rapidly dismutated to hydrogen peroxide. One of the major muscle antioxidants is the glutathione peroxidase/reductase system; by providing a labile pool of reducing equivalents, it is able to consume oxidants and hence protect against oxidative stress. One of the central functions of this system is to degrade peroxides. However, during the ischaemic phase, reduced glutathione is depleted from the myocardium and this antioxidant defence system is therefore compromised. The myocyte contains glutathione peroxidase but relatively little catalase; therefore, loss or impaired function of intracellular antioxidants during ischaemia, as well as depletion of glutathione, predisposes the myocardium to further injury upon reperfusion by reducing the ability of the cell to defend itself against the deleterious effects of radical formation. The intracellular and extracellular sources of reactive oxygen species described above, and the potential delocalization of haem proteins sequestered in an oxidizing locality, may all contribute additively to the myocardial damage due to the ischaemic insult itself. (This is further discussed in Chapter 5.)

Free radicals have been implicated in the pathophysiology of atherosclerosis and myocardial reperfusion injury. This chapter sets the scene for the normal and pathological generation of free radicals and mode of action of antioxidants. The subsequent chapters build on this background to set out the case for the involvement of oxygen-derived free radicals in coronary heart disease.

The author thanks the British Heart Foundation, the British Technology Group, the Ministry of Agriculture, Fisheries and Food, Bioxytech-Paris and Unilever for funding the research programme of her group.

References

1. Aikens, J. and Dix, T. (1991) J. Biol. Chem. **266**, 15091–15098
2. Beck man, J.S., Beckman, T.W., Chen, J., Marshall, P.A. and Freeman, B.A. (1990) Proc. Natl. Acad. Sci. U.S.A. **87**, 1620–1624
3. Beaumont, P., Parsons, B., Deeble, D. and Rice-Evans, C. (eds.) (1989) Free Radicals, Metal Ions and Biopolymers, Richelieu Press, London
4. Biemond, P., Van Eijk, H.G., Swaak, A.J.G. and Koster, J. (1984) J. Clin. Invest. **73**, 1576
5. Biemond, P., Swaak, A.J.G., Van Eijk, H.G. and Koster, J. (1988) Free Radical Biol. Med. **4**, 185–198
6. Koster, J. and Sluiter, W. (1994) in Free Radicals in the Environment, Medicine and Toxicology: Critical Aspects and Current Highlights (Nohl, H., Esterbauer, H. and Rice-Evans, C., eds.), pp. 409–428, Richelieu Press, London
7. Doly, M., Bonhomme, B. and Vennat, J.C. (1986) Opthalmic Res. **18**, 21–27
8. Panter, S.S., Sadrzadeh, S.M., Hallaway, P.E., Haines, P.L., Anderson, V.E. and Eaton, J.W. (1985) J. Exp. Med. **161**, 748–753
9. Yoshino, S., Blake, D.R., Hewitt, S., Morris, C. and Bacon, P.A. (1985) Ann. Rheum. Dis. **44**, 485–490
10. Drexel, H., Dwrozak, E., Kirchmair, W., Milz, M., Puschendorf, B. and Dienstl, F. (1983) Am. Heart J. **105**, 641–651
11. Gutteridge, J.M.C. (1986) FEBS Lett. **201**, 291–295
12. Rice-Evans, C., Okunade, G. and Khan, R. (1989) Free Radical Res. Commun. **7**, 45–54
13. Puppo, A. and Halliwell, B. (1988) Biochem J. **249**, 185–190
14. Rice-Evans, C., Green, E., Paganga, G., Cooper, C. and Wrigglesworth, J. (1993) FEBS Lett. **326**, 177–182
15. Smith, C., Mitchinson, M., Aruoma, O. and Halliwell, B. (1992) Biochem. J. **286**, 901–905
16. Sies, H. (1985) in Oxidative Stress (Sies, H., ed.), pp. 1–8, Academic Press, London,
17. Segal, A.W. and Abo, A. (1993) Trends Biochem. Sci. **18**, 43–47
18. Quie, P.G., White, J.G., Holmes, B. and Good, R.A. (1967) J. Clin. Invest. **46**, 668–679

19. Babior, B.M., Kipnes, R.S. and Curnutte, J.R. (1973) J. Clin. Invest **52**, 741–744
20. Harrison, J. and Schultz, J. (1976) J. Biol. Chem. **251**, 1371–1374
21. Winterbourn, C. (1990) in Oxygen Radicals: Systemic Events in Disease Processes (Das, D. and Essman, W., eds.), pp. 31–70, Karger, U.S.A.
22. Segal, A.W., Geisow, M., Garcia, R., Harper, A. and Miller, R. (1981) Nature (London) **290**, 406–409
23. Segal, A.W., Garcia, R., Godstone, H., Cross, A.R. and Jones, O.T. (1981) Biochem. J. **196**, 363–367
24. Morel, D.W., DiCorleto, P.E. and Chisolm, G. (1984) Arteriosclerosis **4**, 357–364
25. Maly, F.-E., Nakamura, M., Gauchat, J.-F., Urwyler, A., Walker, C., Dahinden, C.A., Cross, A.R. and Jones, O.T.G. (1989) J. Immunol. **142**, 1260–1267
26. Meier, B., Cross, A.R., Hancock, J.T., Kau, F.J. and Jones, O.T.G. (1991) Biochem. J. **275**, 241–245
27. Murrell, G.A.C., Francis, M.J.O. and Bromley, L. (1989) Biochem. Soc. Trans. **17**, 483–484
28. Schraufstatter, I.U. and Jackson, J.H. (1992) in Biological Oxidants: Generation and Injurious Consequences (Cochrane, C.G. and Gimbrone, M.A., eds.), pp. 21–41, Academic Press, New York
29. Blake, D.R., Allen, R. and Lunec, J. (1987) Br. Med. Bull. **43**, 371–385
30. Bellavite, P. (1988) Free Radical Biol. Med. **4**, 225–261
31. Friedl, H.P., Till, G.O., Ryan, U.S. and Ward, P.A. (1989) FASEB J. **3**, 2512–2518
32. McCord, J.M. (1985) N. Engl. J. Med. **312**, 159–163
33. Granger, D.N, Rutili, G. and McCord, J.M. (1981) Gastroenterology **81**, 22–29
34. Kaminski, Z.W., Pohorecki, R., Ballast, C.L. and Domino, E.F. (1986) Circ. Res. **59**, 628–632
35. Ratych, R.E., Chuyknyiska, R.S. and Bulkley, G.B. (1987) Surgery **102**, 122–131
36. Lands, W.E.M. (1979) Annu. Rev. Physiol. **41**, 633–652
37. Kuehl, F., Humes. J., Egan, R., Han, E., Beveridge, G.L. and van Arman, G. (1977) Nature (London) **265**, 270–273
38. Peterson, D.A., Gerrard, J.M., Rao, G.H.R. and White, J.G. (1981) Prog. Lipid Res. **20**, 299–301
39. Smith, W.L. and Marnett, L. (1991) Biochim. Biophys. Acta **1083**, 1–17
40. Marnett, L. and Maddipati, K. (1991) in Peroxidases, Chemistry and Biology (Everse, J., Everse, K. and Grisham, M., eds.), pp. 293–334, CRC Press, New York
41. Ohki, S., Ogino, N., Yamamoto, S. and Hayaishi, O. (1979) J. Biol. Chem. **254**, 829–839
42. Karthein, R., Dietz, R., Nastairiczyle, W. and Ruf, H. (1988) Eur. J. Biochem. **171**, 313–320
43. Ogino, N., Yamamoto, S., Hayaishi, O. and Tokuyama, T. (1979) Biochem. Biophys. Res. Commun. **87**, 184–191
44. Deby, C., Deby-Dupont, G., Noel, F.-X. and Lavergne, L. (1981) Biochem. Pharmacol. **30**, 2243–2249
45. Marnett, L.J. (1984) in Free Radicals in Biology (Pryor, W.A., ed.), pp. 63–94, Academic Press, Orlando
46. Salmon, J.A. (1986) Adv. Drug Res. **15**, 111–167
47. Palmer, R.M.J., Ferrige, A.G and Moncada, S. (1987) Nature (London) **327**, 524–526
48. Marletta, M.A., Tayeh, M.A. and Hevel, J.M. (1990) Biofactors **2**, 219–225
49. Clancy, R.M., Leszczynska-Piziak, J. and Abramson, S.B. (1992) J. Clin. Invest. **90**, 116–1121
50. Ischiropoulos, H., Zhu, L. and Beckman, J.S. (1992) Arch. Biochem. Biophys. **298**, 446–451
51. Radi, R., Beckman, J.W, Bush, K.M. and Freeman, B.A. (1991) Arch. Biochem. Biophys. 481–487
52. Hogg, N., Darley-Usmar, V., Wilson, M.T. and Moncada, S. (1993) FEBS Lett. **326**, 199–203
53. Halliwell, B. (1990) Free Radical Res. Commun. **9**, 1–32
54. Fridovich, I. (1978) Science **201**, 875–880
55. Ogura, Y. and Yamazaki, I. (1983) J. Biochem. **94**, 403–408
56. Cohen, G. and Hochstein, P. (1963) Biochemistry **2**, 1420–1428
57. Cort, W.M. (1982) Adv. Chem. Ser. **200**, 531

58. Bielski, B.H.J and Richter, H.W. (1975) in Antioxidants, Free Radicals and Polyunsaturated Fatty Acids in Biology and Medicine (Diplock, A.T., Gutteridge, J.M.C. and Shukla, U.K.S., eds.), pp 31–40, IFSC, Denmark
59. Cabelli, D.E. and Bielski, B. (1983) J. Phys. Chem. **87**, 1809
60. Nanni, E.J., Stallings, M.D. and Sawyer, D.T. (1980) J. Am. Chem. Soc. **102**, 448
61. Fessenden, R.W. and Varma, N.C. (1978) Biophys. J. **24**, 93
62. Martell, A.E. (1982) Adv. Chem. Ser. **200**, 153
63. Liao, M.-L. and Seib, P. (1987) Food Technol. **41**, 104–111
64. Becker, B.F. (1993) Free Radical Biol. Med. **14**, 615–631
65. Sevanian, A., Davies, K.J.A. and Hochstein, P. (1991) Am. J. Clin. Nutr. **54**, 11295–11345
66. Thomas, M.J. (1992) Free Radical Biol. Med. **12**, 89–91
67. Meadows, J., Smith, R.C. and Reeves, J. (1986) Biochem. Biophys. Res. Commun. **137**, 536–541
68. Cross, C.E., Motchnik, P.A., Bruener, B.A., Jones, D.A., Kaur, H., Ames, B.N. and Halliwell, B. (1992) FEBS Lett. **298**, 269–272
69. Jones, D.A., Kaur, H., Ames, B.N. and Halliwell, B. (1992) FEBS Lett. **298**, 269–278
70. Persky, V.W., Dyer, A.R., Idris-Soven, E., Stamler, J., Shekelle, R.B., Schoenberger, T.A., Berkson, D.M. and Lindberg, H.A. (1979) Circulation **59**, 969–977
71. Brand, F.N., McGee, D.L., Kannel, W.B., Stokes, J. and Castelli, W. (1985) Am. J. Epidemiol. **121**, 1–18
72. Agamah. E.S., Srinivasan, S.R., Webber, L.S. and Berenson, G.S. (1991) J. Lab. Clin. Med. **113**, 241–249
73. Maples, K. and Mason, R. (1988) J. Biol. Chem. **263**, 1709–1712
74. Lam, K.W., Fong, D., Lee. A. and Liu, K.M.D. (1984) J. Inorg. Biochem. **22**, 241–248
75. Stocker, R. and Frei, B. (1991) in Oxidative Stress, Oxidants and Antioxidants (Sies, H., ed), pp. 213–243, Academic Press, London
76. Stocker, R. and Ames, B. (1987) Proc. Natl. Acad. Sci. **84**, 8130–8134
77. Burton, G., Joyce, A. and Ingold, K.U. (1983) Arch. Biochem. Biophys. **221**, 281–290
78. Niki, E., Saito, T., Kawakani, A. and Kamiya, Y. (1984) J. Biol. Chem. **259**, 4177–4182
79. Packer, J.E., Slater, T.F. and Willson, R.L. (1979) Nature (London) **278**, 737–738
80. Scarpa, M., Rigo, A., Maiorino, M., Ursini, F. and Gregolis, C. (1984) Biochim. Biophys. Acta **801**, 215–219
81. Buettner, G. (1993) Arch. Biochem. Biophys. **300**, 535–543
82. Sharma, M.K. and Buettner, G. (1993) Free Radical Biol. Med. **14**, 649–653
83. Bowry, V.W., Ingold, K. and Stocker, R. (1992) Biochem. J. **288**, 341–344
84. Krinsky, N. (1988) Ann. N.Y. Acad. Sci. **551**, 17–33
85. Bendich, A., Olson, J.A. (1989) FASEB J. **3**, 1927–1932
86. Burton, G.W. and Ingold, K.U. (1984) Science **224**, 569–573
87. Di Mascio, P., Kaizer, S. and Sies, H. (1989) Arch. Biochem. Biophys. **274**, 532–538
88. Niki, E. (1993) in Free Radicals and Antioxidants in Nutrition (Corongiu, F., Banni, S., Dessi, M.-A. and Rice-Evans, C., eds.), pp. 13–74, Richelieu Press, London
89. Beyer, R.F. (1990) Free Radical Biol. Med. **8**, 545–565
90. Stocker, R., Bowry, V.W. and Frei, B. (1991) Proc. Natl. Acad. Sci. U.S.A. **88**, 1646–1650
91. Yamamoto, Y., Komuro, E. and Niki, E. (1990) J. Nutr. Sci. Vitaminol. **36**, 505–511
92. Gutteridge, J.M.C., Richmond, R. and Halliwell, B. (1980) FEBS Lett. **112**, 269–272
93. Frei, B., Stocker, R. and Ames, B.N. (1988) Proc. Natl. Acad. Sci. U.S.A. 9748–9752
94. Lentner, C. (ed.) (1984) Geigy Scientific Tables, Vol. 3, CIBA-Geigy, Basel
95. Rice-Evans, C. and Bruckdorfer, K.R. (1992) Mol. Aspects Med. **13**, 1–111
96. Samiec, P.S., Dahm, L.J, Flagg, E.W., Coates, R.J., Eley, J.W. and Jones, D.P. (1993) in Free Radicals and Antioxidants in Nutrition (Corongiu, F., Banni, S., Dessi, M. and Rice-Evans, C., eds.), pp. 269–301, Richelieu Press, London
97. Esterbauer, H., Gebicki, J., Puhl, H. and Jurgens, G. (1992) Free Radical Biol. Med. **13**, 341–390
98. Gey, K.F., Puska, J.M., Jordan, P. and Moser, U.K. (1991) Am. J. Clin. Nutr. **53**, 3265–3345
99. Gaziano, J.M., Manson, J.E., Ridker, P.M., Buring, J.E. and Hennekens, C.H. (1990) Circulation **82** (Suppl. III: 201) Abstract 0796

100. Rimm, E., Stampfer, M.J., Ascherio, A., Giovannucci, E., Colditz, G. and Willett, W. (1993) N. Engl. J. Med. **328**, 1450–1456
101. Stampfer, M.J., Hennekens, C., Manson, J.E., Colditz, G., Robner, G. and Willett, W. (1993) N. Engl. J. Med. **328**, 1444–1449
102. Golumbic, C. and Mattill, H.A. (1941) J. Am. Chem. Soc. **63**, 1279–1280
103. Tappel, A.L. (1968) Geriatrics **23**, 97–105
104. Niki, E., Kawakami, A., Yamamoto, Y. and Kamiya, Y. (1985) Bull. Chem. Soc. Japan **58**, 1971–1975
105. Simic, M. (1990) Methods Enzymol. **186**, 89–100
106. Njus, D. and Kelley, P.M. (1991) FEBS Lett. **284**, 147–151
107. Ernster, L. (1993) in Active Oxygens, Lipid Peroxides and Antioxidants (Yagi, K., ed.), pp. 1–38, CRC Press
108. Tappel, A.L., Brown, W.D., Zolkin, H. and Maier, V.P. (1961) J. Am. Oil Chem. Soc. **38**, 5–9
109. O'Brien, P.J. (1969) Can. J. Biochem. **47**, 485–492
110. Labeque, R. and Marnett, L. (1988) Biochemistry **27**, 7060–7070
111. Roveri, A., Maiorino, M. and Ursini, F. (1994) in Methods in Enzymology, vol. 233 (Packer, L., ed.), pp. 201–212, Academic Press, San Diego
112. Tappel, A.L. and Dillard, C.J. (1981) Fed. Proc. **40**, 174–178
113. Esterbauer, H. (1985) in Free Radicals in Liver Injury (Poli, G., Cheeseman, K., Dianzani, M.U. and Slater, T., eds.), pp. 29–47, IRL Press, Oxford,
114. Sies, H. (1986) Angew. Chemie **25**, 1058–1071
115. Stadtman, E. (1986) Trends Biochem. Sci. **11**, 11–12
116. Stadtman, E.R. (1993) Annu. Rev. Biochem. **62**, 797–821
117. Dean, R. and Davies, M. (1993) Trends Biochem. Sci. **18**, 437–441
118. Rice-Evans, C., Diplock, A.T. and Symons, M.C.R. (1991) Techniques in Free Radical Research, Elsevier Science Publishers, Amsterdam
119. Butler, J., Hoey, B.M. and Lea, J.S. (1988) in Free Radicals, Methodology and Concepts (Rice-Evans, C. and Halliwell, B., eds.), pp 457–459, Richelieu Press, London
120. Grisham, M., Jefferson, M., Melton, D. and Thomas, E. (1984) J. Biol. Chem. **259**, 10404–10413
121. Fliss, H., Weissbach, H. and Brot, N. (1983) Proc. Natl. Acad. Sci. U.S.A. **80**, 7160–7164
122. Cochrane, C.G., Spragg, R.G. and Revak, S.D. (1983) J. Clin. Invest. **71**, 754–761
123. Wolff, S.P., Garner, A. and Dean, R.P. (1986) Trends Biochem. Sci. **11**, 27–31
124. Wolff, S.P. and Dean, R.T (1986) Biochem. J. **234**, 399–403
125. Brown, M.S., Basu, S.K., Falck, J.R., Ho, Y.K. and Goldstein, J.C. (1980) J. Supramol. Struct. **13**, 67–81
126. Haberland, M.E., Olch, C.L. and Fogelman, A.M. (1984) J. Biol. Chem. **259**, 11305–11311
127. Esterbauer, H., Dieber-Rotheneder, M., Waeg, G., Streigl, G. and Jurgens, G. (1990) Chem. Res. Toxicol. **3**, 77–92
128. Hunt, J., Bottoms, M. and Mitchinson, M.J. (1993) Biochem. J. **291**, 529–535
129. Hunt, J.V., Dean, R.T. and Wolff, S.P. (1988) Biochem. J. **256**, 205–212
130. Wolff, S.P. and Dean, R.T. (1987) Biochem. J. **245**, 243–250
131. Hunt, J., Smith, C. and Wolff, J. (1990) Diabetes 39, 1420–1424
132. Hunt, J. (1994) in Free Radicals in the Environment, Medicine and Toxicology: Current Aspects and Critical Highlights (Nohl, H., Esterbauer, H. and Rice-Evans, C., eds.), pp. 137–162, Richelieu Press, London
133. Brownlee, M., Cerami, A. and Vlassara, H. (1988) N. Engl. J. Med. **318**, 1315–1321
134. Jiang, Z.Y., Wolland, A. and Wolff, S.P. (1990) FEBS Lett. **268**, 69–71
135. Marx, G. and Chevion, M. (1986) Biochem. J. **250**, 87–93
136. Eriksson, C.E. and Na, A. (1993) in Free Radicals and Antioxidants in Nutrition (Corongiu, F., Banni, S., Dessi, M.A. and Rice-Evans, C., eds.), pp. 205–224, Richelieu Press, London
137. Lingert, H. and Eriksson, C.E. (1981) Prog. Food Nutr. Sci. **5**, 453
138. Henriksen, T., Mahoney, E.M. and Steinberg, D. (1981) Proc. Natl. Acad. Sci. U.S.A. **78**, 6499–6503
139. Henriksen, T., Mahoney, E.M. and Steinberg, D. (1983) Arteriosclerosis **3**, 149–159
140. Parthasarathy, S., Putz, D.J., Boyd, D., Joy, L. and Steinberg, D. (1986) Arteriosclerosis **26**, 505–510

141. Rankin, S.M. and Leake, D. (1987) Biochem. Soc. Trans. **15**, 485–486
142. Leake, D. and Rankin, S.M. (1990) Biochem. J. **270**, 741–748
143. Paganga, G., Rice-Evans, C., Rule, R. and Leake, D. (1992) FEBS Lett. **303**, 154–158
144. Bourne, L., Collis, C. and Rice-Evans, C. (1994) in Frontiers of Reactive Oxygen Species in Biology and Medicine (Asada, K. and Yoshikama, T., eds.), pp. 469–470, Elsevier Science Publishers, Amsterdam
145. Dee, G., Rice-Evans, C., Obeyesekera, S., Meraji, S., Jacobs, M. and Bruckdorfer, K.R. (1991) FEBS Lett. **294**, 38–42
146. Maiorini, M., Zamburlini, A., Roveri, A. and Ursini, F. (1992) in Dietary Lipids, Antioxidants and the Prevention of Atherosclerosis (Ursini, F., Cadenas, E., eds.), pp. 163–168, Clemp University Publishers, Italy
147. Yla-Herttuala, S., Rosenfeld, M.E., Parthasarathy, S., Glass, C.R., Sigal, E., Witztum, J.L. and Steinberg, D. (1990) Proc. Natl. Acad. Sci. U.S.A. **87**, 6959–6963
148. Morel, D.W., DiCorleto, P.E. and Chisholm, G.M. (1984) Arteriosclerosis **4**, 357–364
149. Heinecke, J.W., Baker, L., Rosen, H. and Chait, A. (1986) J. Clin. Invest. **77**, 757–761
150. Regnstrom, J., Nilsson, J., Tornvall, P., Landou, C. and Harmsten, A. (1992) Lancet **339**, 1183–86
151. Liu, K., Cuddy, T.E. and Pierce, G.N. (1992) Am. Heart. J. **123**, 285–290
152. Andrews, B., Burnand. K., Paganga, G., Browse, N., Rice-Evans, C., Sommerville, K., Leake, D. and Taub, N., (1995) Atherosclerosis **112**, 177–184
153. Omar, B., McCord, J., Downey, J. (1991) in Oxidative Stress, Oxidants and Antioxidants (Sies, H., ed.), pp. 493–527, Academic Press, London
154. Downey, J. (1990). Annu. Rev. Physiol. **52**, 487–504
155. Lucchesi, B. (1990) Annu. Rev. Physiol. **52**, 561–576
156. Buja, L.M., Hagler, H.K. and Willerson, J.T. (1988) Cell Calcium **9**, 205–217
157. Bolli, R., Patel, B.S., Jeroudi, M.O., Lai, E.K. and McCay, P.B. (1988) J. Clin. Invest. **82**, 476–485
158. Bolli, J., Jeroudi, M.O., Patel, B.S., Aruoma, O., Halliwell, B., Lai, E.K. and McKay, P.B. (1989) Circ. Res. **65**, 607–622
159. Ferrari, R., Ceconi, C., Curello, S., Cargnoni, A., Condorelli, E. and Raddino, R. (1985) Vitaminol. Enzymol. **7**, 61–70
160. Shlafer, M., Myers, C.L. and Adkins, S. (1987) J. Mol. Cell Cardiol. **19**, 1195–1206
161. Guanieri, C., Flanigni, F. and Caldarera, C.M. (1980) J. Mol. Cell Cardiol. **12**, 797–808
162. McCord, J.M. (1988) Free Radical Biol. Med. **4**, 9–14
163. Turrens, J.F. and Boveris, A. (1980) Biochem. J. **191**, 421–427

2

Lipid transport and lipoprotein metabolism

M.I. Mackness and P.N. Durrington

University of Manchester Department of Medicine,
Manchester Royal Infirmary, Oxford Road, Manchester M13 9WL, U.K.

Introduction

The impetus for research into lipoproteins in recent years has arisen from their likely relevance to atherosclerotic vascular disease. A primary purpose of the lipoprotein system is to transport lipids, but its theme has undergone a variety of evolutionary variations in different animal species. It is becoming apparent that lipoproteins have wider biological significance than simply lipid transport and are involved in such diverse processes as immune reactions, coagulation and tissue repair [1]. At the same time, it is realized that lipoprotein metabolism may follow very different pathways in different species and that observations made in animals are frequently inapplicable to man. There is thus very often no substitute for clinical studies in man.

The lipoproteins are macromolecular complexes of lipid and protein. Great diversity of composition and physical properties is possible in both health and disease. As such, their classification and definition is particularly difficult. Each lipoprotein has a wide range of components, each with its own metabolic origin and fate (Fig. 1). Lipoprotein components undergo a complex metabolic interplay with receptors, with enzymes located on the lipoproteins and on the capillary endothelium, and with other circulating lipoproteins, both in the vascular compartment and within the tissue fluid space [2,3]. It is thus naïve in the extreme to try to think of serum cholesterol or triglycerides in the same way as serum sodium or glucose, which are transported simply as solutes. The very existence of lipids within the circulation and the tissue fluids is dependent on lipoproteins.

Lipoprotein structure

The general structure of lipoprotein molecules is globular. The physicochemical properties, which govern the arrangement of their constituents, are similar

Fig. 1   The characteristics of the plasma lipoproteins

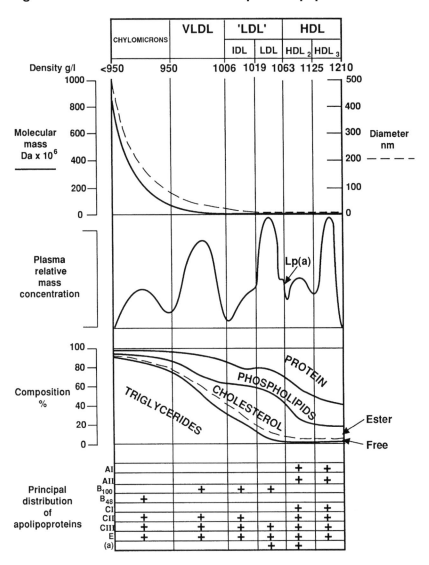

to those involved in the formation of mixed micelles in the lumen of the intestine. Thus, within the outer part of the lipoprotein are found the more-polar lipids, namely the phospholipids and free cholesterol, with their charged groups pointing out towards the water molecules. In physical terms, however, the role of the bile salts, which are also in the outer layer in the mixed micelle, is assumed by proteins, so that the surface of a lipoprotein structurally resembles the outer half of a cell membrane. In the core of the lipoprotein particle are the more hydrophobic lipids, the esterified cholesterol and the triglycerides. These form a central droplet to which the surface coating of phospholipid, cholesterol and protein are anchored by their hydrophobic regions. The exception to this general structure is the newly formed or nascent high-density lipoprotein (HDL), which lacks the central lipid droplet and appears to exist as a disc-like bilayer, consisting largely of phospholipid and protein.

The protein components of lipoproteins are the apolipoproteins, a group of proteins of immense structural diversity. Some of the apolipoproteins have a largely structural role within lipoproteins, while others are major metabolic regulators and some may influence immunological and haemostatic responses apparently unconnected with lipid transport (Table 1). In addition, enzymes are found as components of lipoproteins. The leading example is lecithin–cholesterol acyltransferase (LCAT, EC 2.3.1.43) which is located on HDLs, which are also its site of action. Other enzymes with a less-defined physiological role are also located on HDL, for example, paraoxonase (EC 3.1.8.1), which detoxifies organophosphorous compounds such as nerve gases and pesticides [4].

Lipid transport from the gut to the liver

The products of fat digestion (fatty acids, monoglycerides, lysolecithin and free cholesterol) enter the enterocytes from the mixed micelles. They are re-esterified in the smooth endoplasmic reticulum of these cells. Long-chain fatty acids ($>14C$) are esterified with monoglycerides to form triglycerides and with lysolecithin to form lecithin. Free cholesterol is esterified by the enzyme acyl-CoA : cholesterol O-acyltransferase (ACAT, EC 2.3.1.26). The esterified lipids are then formed into lipoproteins.

The triglycerides, phospholipids and cholesteryl ester are rapidly combined with an apolipoprotein, apo B_{48}, produced in the rough endoplasmic reticulum of the enterocyte. Apo B_{48} is produced by a unique editing process [5,6]. Cells of the gut which produce apo B_{48} contain the full DNA sequence for apolipoprotein B_{100} (apo B_{100}), which has 4704 codons. However, during transcription, a specific enzyme converts a nucleotide in codon 2153 from C to U, thus changing the code for glutamine in apo B_{100} to a

Table 1   Apolipoproteins: their properties and functions

Apolipoprotein	Molecular mass (Da)	Chromosomal location of gene	Plasma concentration (mg/100 ml)	Function
AI	28000	11	6–160	Activation of LCAT Detergent properties
AII	17400	1	20–55	? Activation of hepatic lipase
AIV	44500	11	15	? Lipid transport
B$_{48}$	264000	2	0–2	Secretion of chylomicrons
B$_{100}$	550000	2	60–160	Secretion of VLDL structural protein of LDL Receptor-mediated LDL catabolism
CI	6000	19	3–11	?
CII	8850	19	1–7	Activation of lipoprotein lipase
CIII	8800	11	3–23	? Inhibition of hepatic uptake of chylomicrons and VLDL
D	33000	3	6–10	?
E	34000	19	2–6	Hepatic clearance of chylomicron remnants and IDL Cellular lipoprotein uptake
F	28000	?	2	?
G	72000	?	?	?
H	43000–54000	?	20	?
J	70000	8	10	? Lipid transport ? Membrane chaperone
(a)	300000–700000	6	1–100	? Inhibitor of fibrinolysis Wound repair

Abbreviations used: LCAT, lecithin–cholesterol acyltransferase; VLDL, very-low-density lipoprotein; LDL, low-density lipoprotein; IDL, intermediate-density lipoprotein.

stop codon. An apo B molecule, which has 48% of the molecular mass of apo B_{100}, is therefore produced by the ribosome.

The lipoproteins thus formed, the chylomicrons, are further processed in the Golgi complex, where the apo B_{48} is glycosylated and actively transported to the cell surface for secretion into the lymph (chyle). Chylomicrons are large (>80 nm; density <950 g/l) and rich in triglycerides, but contain only relatively small amounts of protein (Fig. 1). They travel through the lacteals to join the lymph from other parts of the body and enter the blood circulation via the thoracic duct (Fig. 2). In addition to cholesterol absorbed from the diet, they may also receive cholesterol newly synthesized in the gut and cholesterol transferred from other lipoproteins present in the lymph and plasma. The newly secreted or nascent chylomicrons receive C-apolipoproteins from HDLs (which in this respect appear to act as a circulating reservoir, since later in the course of the metabolism of the chylomicron the C-apolipoproteins are transferred back to HDL). The chylomicrons also receive apolipoprotein E (apo E), although the manner in which this happens is unclear. Unlike most other apolipoproteins, which are synthesized either in the liver or gut or both, apo E is exceptional in that it is synthesized (and perhaps secreted) by a large number of tissues (liver, brain, spleen, kidney, lungs and adrenal gland) as well as certain cell types, such as macrophages [3]. In part, the apo E on chylomicrons may come via HDL, but it may also be acquired directly as the chylomicrons circulate through the tissues.

Once the chylomicron has acquired the apolipoprotein, apo CII, it is capable of activating the enzyme lipoprotein lipase (EC 3.1.1.34). This enzyme is attached to heparan sulphate on the luminal surface of the vascular endothelium of tissues with a high requirement for triglycerides, such as skeletal muscle and cardiac muscle (for energy), adipose tissue (for storage) and lactating mammary gland (for milk). Lipoprotein lipase releases triglycerides from the core of the chylomicron by hydrolysing them to fatty acids and glycerol, which are taken up locally by the tissues. In this way the circulating chylomicron becomes progressively smaller. Its triglyceride content decreases and it becomes relatively richer in cholesterol and protein. As the core shrinks, its surface materials (phospholipids, free cholesterol, C-apolipoproteins) become too crowded and there is a net transfer of these to HDL. The cholesteryl-ester-enriched, relatively triglyceride-depleted product of chylomicron metabolism is known as the chylomicron remnant. The apo B_{48}, present from the time of assembly, remains tightly anchored to the core throughout. The apo E also remains and regions of its structure are exposed, which permit catabolism of the chylomicron remnant via the 'remnant receptor' (apo E receptor) of the liver. Remnants are largely removed from the circulation by the liver mediated by the hepatic apo E receptor. Removal of these remnants by the low-density lipoprotein (LDL) receptor (apo B_{100}/E receptors), which can be expressed by virtually every cell in the body, is also possible. However, the

Fig. 2 **An outline of the metabolic pathways for chylo-microns (apolipoprotein B₄₈-containing lipoproteins) secreted by the gut and VLDL (apolipoprotein B₁₀₀-containing lipoproteins) secreted by the liver**

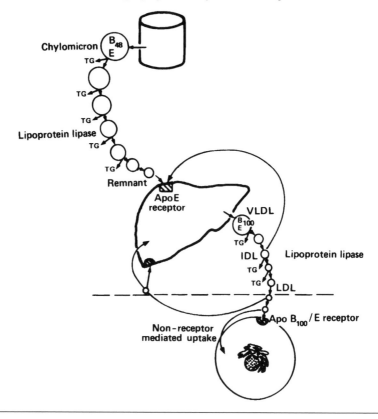

Abbreviations used: B₄₈, apolipoprotein B₄₈; B₁₀₀, apolipoprotein B₁₀₀; E, apolipoprotein E; IDL, intermediate-density lipoprotein; TG, triglycerides.

binding affinity of the hepatic apo E receptor for apo E is greater and chylomicron remnants must compete for binding at the LDL receptor with LDL, the particle concentration of which is much higher than that of the chylomicron remnants (even more so in the tissue fluid than in the plasma). Also, the LDL receptor is rapidly down-regulated by the lysosomal release of free cholesterol into the cell, which follows the entry of lipoprotein–receptor complexes into the cell, whereas expression of the remnant clearance pathway is unaffected by entry of cholesterol into the liver [3].

Lipid transport from the liver to the peripheral tissues

The liver secretes a triglyceride-rich lipoprotein known as very-low-density lipoprotein (VLDL). Teleologically, this allows the supply of triglycerides to tissues in the fasting state as well as postprandially. VLDL particles are somewhat smaller than the chylomicrons (30–80 nm in diameter; density <1006 g/l). Once secreted they undergo exactly the same sequence of changes as chylomicrons; that is the acquisition of C-apolipoproteins and the progressive removal of triglycerides from their core by the enzyme lipoprotein lipase. In man, however, there are some additional metabolic transformations involved in their metabolism, since the liver, unlike the gut, does not esterify cholesterol before its secretion. This is different from species such as the rat. In man, most of the cholesterol released from the liver each day into the circulation is secreted in the VLDL as free cholesterol and it undergoes esterification in the circulation. Free cholesterol is transferred to HDL along a concentration gradient. There it is esterified by the action of the enzyme LCAT, which esterifies the hydroxyl group in the 3-position of cholesterol to a fatty acyl group [7]. This is selectively removed from the 2-position of lecithin to give lysolecithin. The fatty acyl group in this position is generally unsaturated and the cholesteryl ester is thus generally cholesteryl linoleate. Once formed, the cholesteryl ester is transferred back to VLDL. This cannot take place by simple diffusion because cholesteryl ester is intensely hydrophobic and because the concentration gradient is unfavourable. A special protein called cholesteryl ester transfer protein (CETP) or lipid transfer protein is present, which transports cholesteryl ester from HDL to VLDL [8]. It does this in exchange for triglycerides in VLDL and thus also contributes to the removal of core triglycerides from VLDL. The major mechanism for the removal of triglycerides from VLDL is, however, the lipolysis catalysed by lipoprotein lipase.

Another major difference between VLDL and chylomicrons is that the apo B produced by the liver in man is not apo B_{48}, but is almost entirely apo B_{100}. As in the case of chylomicrons, the quantum of apo B packaged in the VLDL remains tightly associated with the particle until its final catabolism, and its amount does not vary after secretion. It is probable that each molecule of VLDL contains one molecule of apo B.

The circulating VLDL particles become progressively smaller as their core is removed by lipolysis and surface materials are transferred to HDL. In normal man, most of the VLDL is converted to smaller LDL particles through the intermediary of a lipoprotein known as intermediate-density lipoprotein (IDL). IDL has a density of 1006–1019 g/l and possesses apo E. In the latter respect it is similar to chylomicron remnants. In some species, such as the rat, it is largely removed by the hepatic apo E receptor and LDL formation is thus bypassed. The enzyme hepatic lipase (EC 3.1.1.3) may be important in the conversion of IDL to LDL. In man, LDL particles, which are relatively enriched in cholesterol, but are small enough (19–25 nm) to cross the vascular endothelium and enter the tissue fluid, serve to deliver cholesterol to the tissues. Their concentration in the extracellular fluid is probably about 10% of that in the plasma. The requirement for cholesterol is for cell membrane repair and growth, and, in the case of specialized tissues such as the adrenal gland, gonads and skin, as a precursor for steroid hormone and vitamin D synthesis.

Human LDL (density 1019–1063 g/l) can be further divided into a spectrum of subfractions (three or five depending on the classification used) which differ in density, molecular mass, size and lipid composition [9]. Many epidemiological studies have indicated that a preponderance of small, dense LDL subfractions is associated with an increased risk of atherosclerosis. An individual's LDL subfraction pattern appears partly to be determined genetically. However, acquired factors may also affect the subclass pattern [10]. Patients with combined hyperlipidaemia display an elevated risk of atherosclerosis and a predominance of small, dense LDL.

The increased atherogenicity of the denser LDL particles may be due to their increased susceptibility to oxidation [11,12]. Some evidence suggests that this susceptibility is due to an increased content of lipids with polyunsaturated fatty acyl groups and a lower content of vitamin E relative to other LDL subfractions [11]. However, the increased oxidizability of the denser LDL particles cannot be entirely explained on that basis [12].

LDL uptake by cells

LDL is able to enter cells by several routes, some of which are regulated according to the cholesterol requirement of each individual cell, some appear to depend almost entirely on the extracellular concentrations of LDL, and some are dependent on modifications of LDL.

The first of these routes is by a cell surface receptor, which specifically binds to lipoproteins that contain apo B_{100} or apo E. This is the LDL receptor (apo B_{100}/E receptor) [13]. As mentioned previously, the receptor, although capable of binding apo E-containing lipoproteins, in most tissues binds largely to apo B_{100}-containing lipoproteins of which LDL is the most widely distributed. After binding, the LDL–receptor complex is internalized within the cell where it undergoes lysosomal degradation (Fig. 3). Its apo B is hydrolysed to its constituent amino acids and its cholesteryl ester is hydrolysed to free cholesterol. The release of this free cholesterol is the signal by which the cellular cholesterol content is precisely regulated by three co-ordinated reactions. First, the enzyme which is rate-limiting for cholesterol biosynthesis (3-hydroxy-3-methylglutaryl-CoA reductase; HMG-CoA reductase; EC 1.1.1.34) is repressed, thus effectively centralizing cholesterol bio-synthesis to organs such as the liver and the gut. Secondly, the synthesis of LDL receptor itself is suppressed. Thirdly, ACAT is activated so that any cholesterol surplus to immediate requirements can be converted to cholesteryl ester, which, because of its hydrophobic nature, forms into droplets within

Fig. 3   The LDL receptor cycle

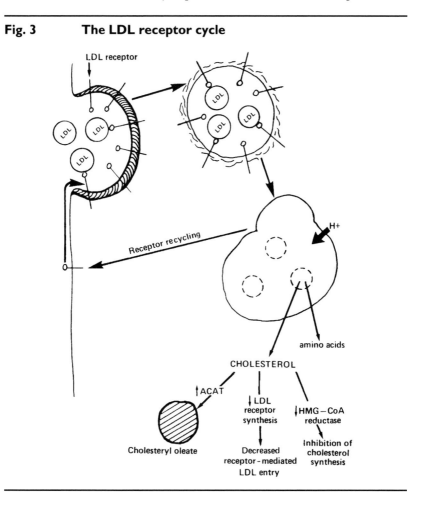

the cytoplasm and is thus conveniently stored [14]. In the liver, the effect of lysosomal release of free cholesterol on the expression of the LDL receptor contrasts with its effect on the hepatic remnant receptor (apo E receptor), which is not subject to any similar regulatory process. It is widely assumed, however, that although free cholesterol released by lysosomal digestion of cholesterol-rich, apo E-containing lipoproteins entering the hepatocyte via the remnant receptor does not influence its own expression, it will, nevertheless, down-regulate the hepatic LDL receptors.

Another major mechanism by which LDL cholesterol may enter the cell is by a non-receptor-mediated pathway. This pathway exists because LDL binds to cell membranes at sites other than those where the LDL receptors are located and some of its cholesterol passes through the membrane. With regard to the structure of LDL, which in many respects is not unlike that of cell membranes, such a phenomenon is perhaps not altogether surprising. HDL is also able to compete with LDL for this type of cell membrane binding [2]. The absence of a receptor means that the binding is of low affinity and thus, at low concentrations, LDL entry by this route may have little significance. However, unlike receptor-mediated entry, non-receptor-mediated LDL uptake is not saturable, but continues to increase with increasing extracellular LDL concentrations. When LDL levels are relatively high, entry of cholesterol into cells by this route may thus assume greater quantitative importance than that via the LDL receptor, which will be both saturated and down-regulated. This appears to be the circumstance in adult man, whose LDL cholesterol is high relative to most animal species and in whom only about one-third of LDL is catabolized by receptors and two-thirds by non-receptor-mediated pathways.

LDL receptor (apo B_{100}/E receptor)

This receptor was first discovered by J.L. Goldstein and M.S. Brown in 1974 (see [14]) when they found that LDL would inhibit cholesterol synthesis in cultured fibroblasts, but HDL would not, and that the inhibitory effect of LDL was absent in fibroblasts from patients who were homozygous for familial hypercholesterolaemia. The gene for the LDL receptor is located on chromosome 19 and contains some 45000 bp, and includes 18 exons (translated sequences) and 18 introns (untranslated intervening sequences). The receptor protein itself contains 839 amino acids. Its apparent molecular mass immediately after synthesis is about 120000 Da, but it subsequently acquires carbohydrate in the Golgi apparatus and undergoes changes in its molecular conformation, altering its electrophoretic mobility, and thus the estimated molecular mass of the mature protein is in the region of 160000 Da. The receptor migrates to the cell surface (Fig. 3), the interval between synthesis and arrival in the coated pit averaging 45 min. There it begins a cycle in which it enters the cell by invagination of coated pits and closure of their necks to form coated endocytic vesicles. These rapidly lose their clathrin coat and fuse to form larger vesicles (endosomes or receptorsomes). ATP-dependent proton pumps in their walls lower the pH of the enclosed fluid and the LDL–receptor complex dissociates. The released LDL receptor leaves the endosome and migrates back to the surface, linking up with other receptors in the coated pit region. The whole cycle is believed to take approximately 10 min.

The LDL receptor undergoes the cycle whether or not it has bound to a lipoprotein, and it is also known that the coated pits contain receptors for other ligands and, therefore, so must the vesicles produced by endocytosis of the coated pits. The endosomes deliver their contents to the lysosomes where LDL undergoes acid hydrolysis. This process is rapid since, when cells in culture are incubated with LDL labelled in its protein moiety with radioactive iodine, the iodine is released into the culture medium within 60 min.

The receptor has at its amino end (first domain) (Fig. 4) the region which binds to apo B and apo E. It contains seven repetitive sequences, each of 40 amino acids. Of these, about seven are cysteine residues, which form disulphide bridges retaining a rigidly cross-linked structure in their part of the molecule. Negatively charged clusters of amino acids are displayed which complement the positively charged receptor binding sites of apo E and apo B.

The binding site region of the receptor molecule is adjacent to a long sequence of amino acids similar to part of the epithelial growth factor (EGF) precursor. It should be noted that there is no similarity with the portion of EGF released. Thus, although the similarity may be informative about how different proteins have evolved, it does not suggest that there is a functional link between the two proteins. The same is probably true of the sequences in the receptor binding part of the molecule which have similarities with the C9 component of complement.

The next sequence of amino acids is rich in sugar and this leads on to a hydrophobic region of the molecule, which spans the cell membrane. The final carboxyl end of the molecule extends into the cytoplasm and its interaction with clathrin is essential for the arrival of the receptor in the coated pit region of the cell membrane.

The chylomicron remnant receptor (apo E receptor)

The great problem with the chylomicron receptor concept has been the failure to isolate it and perform the definitive experiments that have been possible with the LDL receptor.

The question thus arises as to whether the LDL receptor and the chylomicron remnant receptor are one and the same. However, in patients homozygous for familial hypercholesterolaemia only small increases in IDL occur and their clearance of chylomicron remnants is relatively normal, particularly if compared with patients with type III hyperlipoproteinaemia in whom polymorphism or mutation of apo E decreases receptor binding. This argues very much for there being a second receptor for chylomicron remnants which is unaffected by the LDL receptor mutation and which has the capacity to

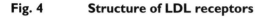

Fig. 4   Structure of LDL receptors

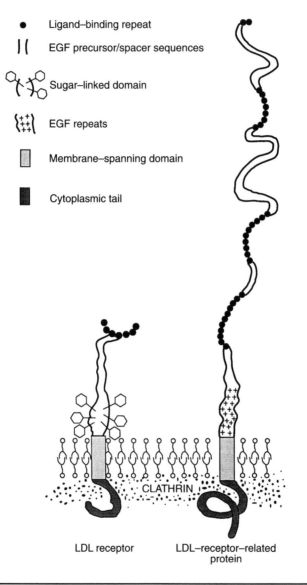

- Ligand–binding repeat

| (EGF precursor/spacer sequences

Sugar–linked domain

{+++} EGF repeats

Membrane–spanning domain

Cytoplasmic tail

CLATHRIN

LDL receptor   LDL–receptor–related
                      protein

catabolize chylomicron remnants, including those which would normally be removed by the LDL receptor.

The most likely candidate for the chylomicron receptor is another recently discovered member of the LDL supergene family termed the LDL-receptor-related protein (LRP) (Fig. 4). This is an enormous protein of 4525 amino acids with an initial molecular mass of 600 000 Da which after proteolytic shortening in the Golgi complex, appears as a membrane receptor with a molecular mass of 515 000 Da [15].

The LRP resembles four LDL receptors joined together. Instead of a single, negatively charged, ligand-binding domain, consisting of seven cysteine-rich repeats homologous to complement situated at its amino end, LRP has four of these ligand-binding sites. One at the amino terminal end has two cysteine-rich repeats. Three others are then strung out along the molecule consisting of 8, 10 and 11 cysteine-rich repeats, respectively. In between the ligand-binding sites are sequences resembling the EGF precursor. LRP lacks the sugar-rich domain of the LDL receptor. Instead, a sequence more closely resembling EGF itself links it to its hydrophobic, membrane-spanning region. This in turn leads to a cytoplasmic tail. Like that of the LDL receptor this anchors the molecule to the clathrin of the coated pit region of the cellular membrane; however, in the case of the LRP it is twice as long, perhaps because its size demands a more secure anchorage. LRP appears to undergo a similar recycling process to LDL. LRP and the LDL receptor are part of a family of molecules with certain features in common which have evolved from a common ancestral gene, which includes the vitellogenin receptor of egg-laying birds and reptiles and glycoprotein 330, the function of which is unknown, but which is the antigen for an autoimmune nephritis in rats.

Brown *et al.* [15] first suggested in 1988 that the LRP was the chylomicron receptor. At the time of writing there is a good case for this, but it is not proven. The LRP is found in a wide variety of tissues and cultured cells, yet chylomicron remnant catabolism is targeted to the liver. Perhaps the fenestrated capillary endothelium of the liver means that the large chylomicron remnant particles come into contact with hepatocytes, whereas they less readily cross other vascular endothelia to come into contact with other cell types. Perhaps also the liver showers the remnants with apo E during their passage through it, thus enhancing LRP binding, or maybe it has some trapping mechanism, possibly involving extracellular glycosaminoglycans or hepatic lipase.

LRP is certainly not a receptor dedicated to the clearance of lipoproteins. It has a major function in clearing α_2-macroglobulin from the circulation. This is a protein which scavenges serine proteases and certain growth factors and cytokines leaking into the plasma compartment. The LRP also appears to bind other molecules, such as lipoprotein lipase and plasminogen activator/plasminogen activator inhibitor complexes. Not all the ligands binding to LRP compete with each other, suggesting that the ligand-binding sites may each be specific for different molecular complexes. However, a receptor-associated protein, which can competitively block all ligand binding, has been identified.

Other receptors for apo B-containing lipoproteins

Other receptors for apo E- and apo B-containing lipoproteins undoubtedly exist. Two families of these present on the macrophage have excited considerable interest, because, although their contribution to LDL catabolism may not be great, they may lie at the heart of atherogenesis. They are the β-VLDL receptor and acetyl-LDL receptor. Uptake at both these receptors *in vitro* is so rapid (and not down-regulated) that foam cells resembling those in arterial fatty streaks are formed (see Chapter 5 by Jessup and Leake).

In vitro, the β-VLDL receptor allows the uptake of lipoproteins with a density less than 1006 g/l (a mixture of apo E-rich chylomicron remnants and IDL) from patients with type III hyperlipoproteinaemia [16] and perhaps also VLDL and IDL from diabetic subjects. Recently, studies utilizing human monocyte-derived macrophages have suggested that the mechanism for VLDL receptor clearance by the macrophage is via the LDL receptor. Lipoprotein lipase on the macrophage outer surface facilitates the binding of VLDL and β-VLDL to proteoglycans and the enzyme begins the process of lipolysis of the VLDL. Apo E secreted by the macrophages may be incorporated into VLDL (β-VLDL is already rich in apo E). Both processes alter the affinity of VLDL for the macrophage-LDL receptor, facilitating the receptor-mediated uptake of VLDL. Lipoprotein lipase has also been shown to enhance LDL binding and uptake by both cultured fibroblasts and macrophages.

The acetyl-LDL and oxidized-LDL receptors permit the rapid uptake by macrophages in tissue culture of LDL modified, for example, by oxidation [17,18]. The uptake of unmodified LDL by the macrophage via the LDL receptor is too slow for foam cell formation and is even slower than for other cell types, such as fibroblasts. It is now known that macrophages have more than one type of receptor for oxidized LDL [19]. Although these receptors were first discovered because oxidized LDL competed for uptake with LDL modified by acetylation, the competition is incomplete and receptors for oxidized LDL other than the acetyl-LDL receptor have been reported. The macrophage acetyl-LDL receptor is also responsible for the uptake of LDL–proteoglycan complexes [20]; it is frequently referred to as the scavenger receptor. It is increasingly common for the whole family of receptors capable of taking up oxidatively modified LDL to be called oxidized-LDL receptors.

Reverse cholesterol transport

In man, cholesterol is transported from the gut and liver in quantities that greatly exceed its conversion to steroid hormones and its loss through the skin in sebum. Therefore, except when the requirement for membrane synthesis is high, for example during growth or active tissue repair, the greater part of the cholesterol transported to the tissue (if it is not to accumulate there) must be returned to the liver for elimination in the bile, or for reassembly into lipoproteins. The return of cholesterol from the tissues to the liver is termed 'reverse cholesterol transport' (Fig. 5). It is less well understood than the pathways by which cholesterol reaches the tissues, but it may well be critical to the development of atheroma. HDL has many features which make it very likely that it is intimately involved in the reverse transport process.

The precursors of plasma HDL (nascent) are small (<0.45 nm) lipoprotein particles composed largely of protein and phospholipid secreted mainly by the gut and the liver, probably as disc-shaped bilayers. In the circulation, the smallest HDL particles are termed pre-β-HDLs because of their electrophoretic mobility. This pre-β-HDL may be derived from the nascent HDL secreted from the liver and gut, but may also in part be regenerated from the metabolism of larger HDL particles. Pre-β-HDL is released during the lipolysis of triglyceride-rich lipoproteins [21,22]. It may represent nascent HDL travelling loosely attached to the triglyceride-rich lipoproteins to prevent its filtration through the renal glomeruli. This mechanism for its release also maximizes its concentration in tissue where lipoprotein catabolism is active.

Apolipoprotein AI constitutes the major protein component of nascent and pre-β-HDLs and their other major component is phospholipids. Other apolipoproteins present in HDL and the bulk of its lipid are acquired as it circulates through the vascular and other extracellular fluids. In this respect, the transformation of HDL from its lipid-poor precursor to a relatively lipid-rich molecule is the opposite to that which the other lipoproteins undergo following their secretion.

HDL is a small particle compared with the other lipoproteins (0.45–19 nm) and easily crosses the vascular endothelium so that its concentration in the tissue fluids is much closer to its intravascular concentration than is the case for LDL [23]. Because the serum HDL cholesterol concentration is only about one-fifth that of the LDL cholesterol concentration, it is often wrongly assumed that its particle concentration is lower. In fact, the particle concentrations of HDL and LDL in human plasma are often similar, and in the tissue fluids there are several times as many HDL molecules as those of other lipoproteins present unless capillaries have a fenestrated endothelium. Thus the cells are in contact with higher concentrations of HDL molecules than of any other lipoprotein. In man, unlike the rat, HDL serves no apparent function in transporting cholesterol to cells.

Both aqueous diffusion and an HDL receptor have been suggested to explain cholesterol efflux from cells to HDL. In the aqueous diffusion model [24], free cholesterol desorbs from both cell membranes and HDL into the aqueous phase between them. The cholesterol is then rapidly reabsorbed by

Fig. 5   **The pathways by which cholesterol may be returned to the liver from the tissues**

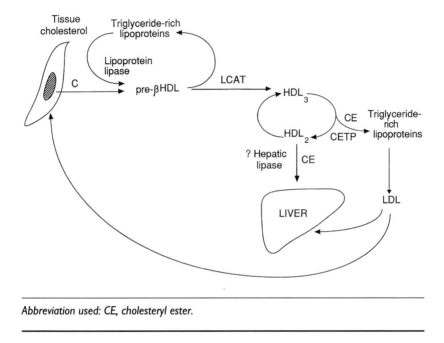

Abbreviation used: CE, cholesteryl ester.

either HDL or the cells. Thus, it is suggested, there is an equilibrium determined by factors driving the reabsorption in one direction or the other. Several factors are in fact present which favour the transfer of free cholesterol from cells to HDL. The phospholipid content of HDL directly influences the rate of cholesterol efflux. Depleting HDL of its phospholipids reduces the amount of cholesterol it can acquire [24]. Thus the phospholipid-rich pre-β-HDL is a likely initial acceptor of cellular free cholesterol. Its candidature for this role is further strengthened because the LCAT on pre-β-HDL is particularly active [21]. Free cholesterol entering pre-β-HDL is thus esterified and moves into the core of the lipoprotein because of its increased hydrophobicity compared with free cholesterol. This decreases the free cholesterol content at the surface of the particle, re-establishing a gradient favourable for free cholesterol uptake by pre-β-HDL. Some evidence also suggests that cells in tissue culture express receptors for HDL, particularly HDL$_3$ which might permit the transfer of cholesterol out of the cell [25]. However, the passage of cholesterol across the cell membrane may not simply depend on receptors, since cholesterol must first be unesterified (unless CETP can cross the cell membrane to bind with it, which is unlikely, or possibly apo E or apo J synthesized within certain cells transport it out). Factors regulating the intracellular cholesterol esterase activity to release free cholesterol may also be important in determining the amount of cholesterol available to be transported out of the cell [1].

Cholesterol cannot simply be taken up by pre-β-HDL, esterified and packed into its core (converting it to HDL_3 and HDL_2 which are then cleared by the liver), because LDL equivalent to 1500 mg of cholesterol is catabolized each day, whereas the rate of catabolism of the HDL apolipoproteins AI and AII would permit less than 200 mg of HDL cholesterol to be catabolized each day. Therefore, (i) the liver must be capable of selectively removing cholesterol from HDL and then returning the particle to the circulation with most of its apolipoprotein intact, or (ii) the cholesterol in HDL must be transferred to another lipoprotein class which is capable of being cleared in quantity by the liver, or (iii) a class of HDL which contains little apo AI or AII must be cleared by the liver at a much greater rate than the bulk of HDL.

In support of (i), there is some evidence that hepatic lipase might act on the phospholipid envelope of HDL during its passage through hepatic sinusoids and release the cholesteryl ester contained in its core, and that some hepatic trapping or even receptor-mediated mechanism might enhance the process. On the other hand, in support of (ii), there is a well-established mechanism for the transfer of cholesteryl ester from HDL to VLDL and LDL through the agency of CETP. Once on VLDL, the cholesteryl ester can then arrive at the liver via the binding of IDL to the remnant receptor, or when LDL enters the liver after binding to the LDL receptor or by the non-receptor-mediated route. This mechanism may, however, also have a downside; cholesteryl ester transferred from HDL to lower density lipoproteins may enter the LDL, which is an atherogenic lipoprotein. There is an increase in cholesteryl ester transfer from HDL to VLDL/LDL in people with low HDL levels and hypertriglyceridaemia [26], with established coronary artery disease [27] and with diabetes mellitus [28]. Evidence for pathway (iii), the return of cholesterol to the liver from HDL by a rapidly metabolized form of HDL present at low concentration in serum, is at present largely lacking.

It is incorrect to regard HDL as a single homogeneous species, since it is known to be a mixture of particles which differ in size, in lipid and apolipoprotein composition and in function. Two peaks of HDL are seen in the analytical ultracentrifuge; the less-dense peak is designated HDL_2 (density = 1063–1125 g/l) and the more-dense peak, HDL_3, (density = 1125–1210 g/l). HDL_3 may be converted to HDL_2 by the acquisition of cholesterol, HDL_3 thus being a precursor form of HDL_2. Whereas antisera to apo AI precipitate virtually all of HDL, antisera to AII do not, suggesting that some molecules of HDL contain AI and AII, whereas others contain AI only. The AI-only HDL molecules which predominate in HDL_2 may arise from very different metabolic channels from the AI/AII particles. Furthermore, HDL may contain other molecular species with overlapping density ranges, such as lipoprotein(a) [Lp(a)]. HDL thus represents a rather heterogeneous entity.

Lipoproteins and atherosclerosis

In prospective epidemiological studies, the serum HDL cholesterol level is inversely associated with the risk of coronary heart disease (CHD), whereas the association with LDL-cholesterol is positive [1]. Most of this book is devoted to how LDL may be involved in atherogenesis. Therefore, this will not be considered further here. Why HDL apparently protects against CHD may, however, be an equally important question since, in women and the elderly, low HDL is a more potent risk factor than high LDL. It has been proposed that HDL exerts its protective effect because of its role in reverse cholesterol transport discussed previously. Recently an additional mechanism has become apparent. HDL has been shown to inhibit LDL oxidation by both redox metals and arterial cells in culture [29]. Our own findings suggest that HDL acts to prevent the formation of lipid peroxides in LDL when they are both incubated under oxidizing conditions [30]. Its effect may be greater than that of the fat-soluble vitamins.

Preliminary studies have indicated that the mechanism whereby HDL prevents LDL oxidation is enzymic and at least part of the protection can be ascribed to the presence of the enzyme paraoxonase on HDL [31]. HDL has associated with it a number of enzymes other than LCAT and paraoxonase, such as a phospholipase and a serine protease whose metabolic roles are obscure, but they also may be relevant to the ability of HDL to inhibit LDL-peroxide accumulation. The physiological generation of lysolecithin in huge quantities on HDL as a result of the action of the enzyme LCAT during cholesterol esterification may mean that systems have evolved on HDL to dispose of this cytotoxic substance (which is also generated on LDL after oxidation). The presence of HDL at relatively high concentrations in the interstitial fluid may also mean it has wider relevance in preventing the accumulation of lipid peroxides in tissues other than the arterial wall, which requires further study.

Lp(a)

Lp(a) is a lipoprotein with a density in the range 1030–1100 g/l which thus overlaps with LDL and HDL_2. The protein moiety of Lp(a) in common with LDL contains one molecule of apo B, but in addition there is a molecule of another huge apolipoprotein termed apolipoprotein (a) [apo(a)] (Fig. 6). Apo(a) has a domain which is largely identical to the protease domain of plasminogen, but which cannot be activated to promote fibrinolysis. Plasminogen has a finger-like process comprising five kringles (compressed loops with internal disulphide bridges resembling pretzels). In apo(a), kringle 5 is preserved but kringle 4 is repeated many times and kringles 1–3 are absent. There is considerable variation in the molecular mass of apo(a) (between 300 000 and 700 000 Da), the isoforms arising due to differences in the number of kringle 4s, which is determined at a single allele on chromosome 6 so that an individ-

Fig. 6   **The structures of Lp(a) and plasminogen**

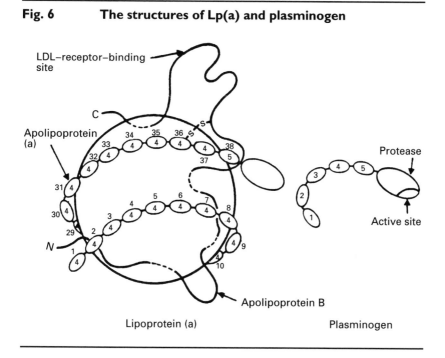

Lipoprotein (a)   Plasminogen

ual expresses one or two of the isoforms. The circulating concentration of Lp(a) is inversely related to the molecular mass of the isoforms [32].

The serum Lp(a) concentration is related to the risk of developing CHD and cerebral arteriosclerosis. It has been extracted from atheromatous plaques and, indeed, may be more likely to be retained in the arterial sub-intima than LDL because it adheres to glycosaminoglycans and to fibrin, and in tissue culture will also bind to plasminogen receptors on macrophages. This may therefore increase the likelihood that it will be oxidized and taken up by macrophages to form foam cells, and Lp(a) may thus contribute relatively more to atherogenesis than LDL [32,33]. Its levels are particularly high in familial hypercholesterolaemia and renal disease. It might also have a role in myocardial and cerebral infarction by promoting thrombosis through interfering in thrombolysis [32]. Currently, much of what is known about Lp(a) in relation to atherogenesis is speculative and any explanation must take into account its higher concentration in Black as opposed to White people, despite the relatively lower rates of CHD in Black people.

References

1. Durrington, P.N. (1994) Hyperlipidaemia: Diagnosis and Management, 2nd edn., Butterworth Heinemann, Oxford
2. Karathanasis, S.K. (1992) in Molecular Genetics of Coronary Artery Disease: Candidate Genes and Processes in Atherosclerosis (Lusis, A.J., Rotter, J.I. and Sparkes, R.S., eds.), pp. 140–171, Karger, Basel
3. Schumaker, V. and Lembertas, A. (1992) in Molecular Genetics of Coronary Artery Disease: Candidate Genes and Processes in Atherosclerosis (Lusis, A.J., Rotter, J.I. and Sparkes, R.S., eds.), pp. 98–139, Karger, Basel
4. Mackness, M.I. (1989) Biochem. Pharmacol. **38**, 385–390
5. Powell, L.M., Wallis, S.C., Pease, R.J., Edwards, Y.H., Knott, T.J. and Scott, J. (1987) Cell **50**, 831–840
6. Chen, S-H., Habib, G., Yang, C.Y., Gu, Z-W., Lee, B.R., Weng, S., Silberman, S.R., Cai, S.J., Deslypere, J.P., Rosseneu, M., et al. (1987) Science **283**, 363–366
7. Gillett, M.P.T. and Owen, J.S. (1992) in Lipoprotein Analysis — A Practical Approach (Converse, C.A. and Skinner, E.R., eds.), pp. 187–202, Oxford University Press, Oxford
8. Rye, K-A. and Barter, P.J (1992) in Structure and Function of Apolipoproteins (Rosseneu, M. ed.), pp. 401–426, CRC Press, Boca Raton
9. Krauss, R.M. (1991) Curr. Opin. Lipidol. **2**, 248–252
10. Campos, H., Blijlevens, E., McNamara, J.R., Ordovas, J.M., Posner, B.M., Wilson, P.W., Castelli, W.P. and Schaefer, F.J (1992) Arteriosclerosis Thrombosis **12**, 1410–1419
11. De Graaf, J., Hak-Lemmers, H.L.M., Hectors, M.P.C., DeMacker, P.N.M., Mendricks, J.C.M. and Stalenhoef, A.F.M. (1991) Arteriosclerosis Thrombosis **11**, 298–306
12. Dejager, S., Bruckert, E. and Chapman, M.J. (1993) J. Lipid Res. **34**, 295–308
13. Coetzee, G.A. and van de Westhuyzen, D.R. (1992) Curr. Opin. Lipidol. **3**, 60–61
14. Brown, M.S. and Goldstein, J.L. (1986) Science **232**, 34–47
15. Brown, M.S., Herz, J., Kowal, R.C. and Goldstein, J.L. (1991) Curr. Opin. Lipidol. **2**, 65–72
16. Hussain, M.M., Maxfield, F.R., Mas-Oliva, J., Tabas, I., Ji, Z.S., Innerarity, T.L. and Mahley, R.W. (1991) J. Biol. Chem. **266**, 13936–13940
17. Keidur, S., Kaplan, M., Rosenblat, M., Brook, G.J. and Aviram, M. (1992) Metabolism **41**, 1185–1192
18. Ramsey, S.C., Obunike, J.C., Arad, Y., Deckelbaum, R.J. and Goldberg, I.J. (1992) J. Clin. Invest. **90**, 1504–1512
19. Sparrow, C.P., Parthasarathy, S. and Steinberg, D. (1989) J. Biol. Chem. **264**, 2599–2604
20. Vijayagopal, P., Srinivasan, S.R., Radhakrishnamurthy, B. and Berenson, G.S. (1993) Biochem. J. **289**, 837–844
21. Neary, R., Bhatnagar, D., Durrington, P.N., Ishola, M., Arrol, S. and Mackness, M.I. (1992) Atherosclerosis **89**, 35–48
22. Kunitake, S.T., Mendel, C.M. and Hennessy, I.K. (1992) J. Lipid Res. **33**, 1807–1816
23. Eisenberg, S. (1984) J. Lipid Res. **25**, 1017–1058
24. Rothblat, G.H., Mehlberg, F.H., Johnson, W.J. and Phillips, M.C. (1992) J. Lipid Res. **33**, 1901–1908
25. Slotte, J.P., Oram, J.F. and Bierman, E.L. (1987) J. Biol. Chem. **262**, 12904–12907
26. Bhatnagar, D., Durrington, P.N., Mackness, M.I., Arrol, S., Winocour, P.H. and Prais, H. (1992) Atherosclerosis **92**, 49–57
27. Bhatnagar, D., Durrington, P.N., Channon, K.M., Prais, H. and Mackness, M.I. (1992) Atherosclerosis **98**, 25–32
28. Bhatnagar, D., Durrington, P.N., Kumar, S., Young, C., Winocour, P.H., Prais, H. and Mackness, M.I. (1992) Diabetic Med. **9** (Suppl. 2), S16
29. Mackness, M.I., Arrol, S., Abbott, C.A. and Durrington, P.N. (1993) Chemico-Biological Interactions **87**, 161–171
30. Mackness, M.I., Abbott, C.A., Arrol, S. and Durrington, P.N. (1993) Biochem. J. **294**, 829–834

31. Mackness, M.I., Arrol, S., Abbott, C.A. and Durrington, P.N. (1993) Atherosclerosis **104**, 129–135

32. MBewu, A.D. and Durrington, P.N. (1990) Atherosclerosis **85**, 1–14

33. Beisiegel, U. (1991) Curr. Opin. Lipidol. **2**, 317–323

3

The chemistry of oxidation of lipoproteins

Hermann Esterbauer

Institute of Biochemistry, University of Graz, Schubertstr. 1, A-8010 Graz, Austria

Introduction

The last decades saw a series of remarkable studies suggesting that oxidation of low-density lipoprotein (LDL) might be a risk factor in atherosclerosis. Many reviews published in journals [1–10] and books [11–13] reflect the considerable interest in this new concept. Early atherosclerotic lesions are characterized by massive accumulation of lipid-laden foam cells in the sub-endothelial space of arteries. Most of the foam cells are derived from monocyte-macrophages, and much of the interest in oxidized LDL (oLDL) stems from the discovery that it exhibits properties *in vitro* which could explain the immigration of monocytes into the arterial wall, their differentiation into resident macrophages and the conversion to foam cells. Most significant in this respect is the fact that oLDL bypasses the normal tight control exercised by the classical LDL receptor, but is avidly endocytosed via a scavenger receptor pathway of macrophages. It may also be very significant that oLDL contains highly cytotoxic lipid peroxidation products; the release of such diffusible toxins from oLDL deposited in the arterial wall would be a constant irritant for the endothelial cell layer and provoke a number of other deleterious effects, such as endothelial cell death, platelet aggregation, release of growth factors, disturbance of eicosanoid homoeostasis, accumulation of inflammatory cells and increased infiltration of LDL. Inhibition by oLDL of endothelium-derived relaxing factor (EDRF)-mediated relaxation of smooth muscle cells, the immunogenicity of oLDL, and the stimulation (preferentially by minimally oxidized LDL) of endothelial cells to release a number of biologically active factors [monocyte chemotactic proteins, endothelial leucocyte adhesion molecules (ELAMS), growth factors for monocytes] also support the hypothesis that the atherogenicity of LDL increases when it becomes oxidized.

Furthermore, it has been suggested that oLDL may activate T-lymphocytes in atherosclerotic lesions [14] and stimulate proliferation of smooth muscle cells by inducing expression of the gene coding for the A-chain of platelet-derived growth factor [15]. Taken together, these data on the functional and biological properties of oLDL strongly support the hypothesis of its atherogenic role.

LDL oxidation can be initiated *in vitro* by incubating it with macrophages, endothelial cells, smooth muscle cells and lymphocytes, or in cell-free systems utilizing a variety of pro-oxidants such as lipoxygenase, myeloperoxidase, defined oxygen radicals, u.v.-light, γ-irradiation, haem, copper ions, hypochlorous acid and others. Traces of transition metals, in free form or in redox-active complexes, are generally agreed to be essential for producing oLDL with the properties described above. The mechanism of initiation and progression of LDL oxidation *in vivo* is largely a matter of speculation. It is thought to occur not in the circulation but within the arterial wall itself, where LDL is sequestered by proteoglycans and other extracellular matrix constituents [2,12]. LDL isolated from the arterial wall shares some functional and biological properties with LDL oxidized *in vitro* [7].

It is one thing to demonstrate the biological properties of oLDL, but quite another to study the complex chemistry of LDL oxidation and to analyse the structure of the large number of oxidation products. This topic, although of central importance for the oxidation hypothesis, has not yet received the broad attention it deserves.

Oxidation of LDL is a lipid peroxidation chain reaction driven by free radicals. LDL oxidation therefore possesses the general characteristics of lipid peroxidation reactions and free radical reactions. What makes the process and its dynamics so complex is the fact that all components of LDL, i.e. antioxidants, phospholipids, cholesteryl ester, triglycerides and apolipoprotein B (apo B), participate at certain stages leading to multiple secondary and tertiary reactions.

This chapter will focus mainly on the composition of native LDL and LDL oxidized by copper ions.

Composition of native LDL

Human LDL is defined as the population of lipoproteins which can be isolated from plasma by ultracentrifugation within a density gradient of 1019–1063 g/l. LDL molecules are large spherical particles with a diameter of 19–25 nm and a molecular mass of 1.8–2.8 million Da (average 2.5 million Da). The mean chemical composition (% by weight) deduced from various reports (for a review, see [7]) is 22.3% phospholipid, 5.9% triglyceride, 9.6% free cholesterol, 42.2% cholesteryl ester and 22.0% protein. The lipid and fatty acid composition is shown in Table 1. The mean total cholesterol content is 34.7%. Based on a molecular mass of 2.5 million Da, each LDL

Table 1   Lipid composition and individual fatty acids in native LDL

	Lipid composition		
	(nmol/mg of LDL protein)		(mol/mol of LDL)
	Mean	±S.D.	Mean
Total phospholipids	1300	±227	700
Phosphatidylcholine	818	—	450
Phosphatidylethanolamine	19	—	10
Lysophosphatidylcholine	30	—	16
Sphingomyelin	336	—	185
Ethanolamine plasmalogen	43	—	24
Choline plasmalogen	4	—	2
Triglycerides	304	±140	170
Free cholesterol	1130	±82	600
Cholesteryl ester	2960	±220	1600
Total cholesterol	4090	—	2200
Free fatty acids	48	—	26
Palmitic acid	1260	±375	693
Palmitoleic acid	80	±44	44
Stearic acid	260	±118	143
Oleic acid	825	±298	454
Linoleic acid	2000	±541	1100
Arachidonic acid	278	±100	153
Docosahexaenoic acid	53	±31	29
Total fatty acids	4756	—	2616
Total PUFAs	2330	—	1280

Lysophosphatidylcholine value taken from [16], phosphatidylethanolamine and plasmalogen values taken from [17], all others taken from [7].

particle would contain about 1600 molecules of cholesteryl ester and 170 molecules of triglyceride, which form a central lipophilic core. The core is surrounded by a monolayer of about 700 molecules of phospholipid and 600 molecules of free cholesterol. The main phospholipids are phosphatidylcholine (63%) and sphingomyelin (26%). The plasmalogen content may be important for the oxidation resistance of LDL, particularly ethanolamine plasmalogen which has been reported to act as an antioxidant [18]. The total amount of fatty acids in an LDL molecule is approx. 2600 and about half of these are polyunsaturated fatty acids (86% linoleic acid 18:2, 12% arachidonic acid 20:4, 2% tocosahexaenoic acid 22:5). The standard deviations in Table 1 indicate a rather strong variation in fatty acid distribution, which might be significant for the variation in the oxidation resistance of LDL.

The antioxidants contained in LDL are listed in Table 2. On a molar base, by far the most abundant is α-tocopherol, the amount of 11.58 nmol/mg of protein equals about 6 molecules per LDL particle. Ethanolamine plasmalogen amounts to 24 molecules per LDL particle, but it remains to be determined whether it shows chain-breaking antioxidant activity in LDL. All other compounds with potential antioxidant activity are present in much smaller amounts than α-tocopherol. In our analyses, ubiquinol-10, with 0.1 molecule per LDL particle, is only a minor antioxidant. Stocker et al. [19] showed that ubiquinol-10 amounts to only 3.5% of α-tocopherol (the concentrations given for native LDL were 1.2 μM ubiquinol-10 and 36 μM α-tocopherol). That would mean 0.2 molecules per LDL particle, based on an α-tocopherol value of 6 molecules per LDL particle. In a later study [20], the same group reported that 0.5–1.0 molecules of ubiquinol-10 are present per LDL particle. Eighty-five percent of ubiquinol-10 is in the reduced form.

An excellent article by Yang and Pownall [21] reviewed the structure and function of the apo B of LDL. Apo B is one of the largest known monomeric proteins, the single polypeptide chain contains 4536 amino acids, and the calculated molecular mass is 512.937 Da. The number of amino acid residues per apo B are Ala, 266; Asp + Asn, 478; Arg, 148; Cys, 25; Glu + Gln, 529; Gly, 207; His, 115; Ile, 288; Leu, 523; Lys, 356; Met, 78; Phe, 223; Pro, 169; Ser, 393; Thr, 298; Trp, 37; Tyr, 152 and Val, 251. The apo B is glycosylated and the carbohydrate content can amount to 9–10 % (by weight) of apo B, with galactose, mannose, N-acetylglucosamine and sialic acid residues. Camejo et al. [22] reported that the sialic acid content is important for the sequestering of LDL by proteoglycans in the arterial wall. From the 25 cysteine residues, seven probably have the free sulphydryl group, whereas the rest form disulphide bonds, and two of the sulphydryl groups are exposed to the LDL surface. These may play a role in the reductive activation of transition metal ions, e.g. $Cu^{2+} + RSH \rightarrow Cu^{+} + \frac{1}{2}RSSR$.

Finally, it is important to note that LDL with the buoyant density 1019–1063 g/l, consists of subfractions differing in size, molecular mass, density and composition [7,23]. About 75% of individuals belong to phenotype A, characterized by an LDL profile with a predominance of larger and less-dense (1025–1038 g/l) LDL. Individuals with phenotype B (about 25% of the population) have an LDL profile with a predominance of smaller, dense (>1038 g/l) LDL. Epidemiological studies have shown that phenotype B is

Table 2   Antioxidants in native LDL

	Antioxidant composition		
	(nmol/mg of LDL protein)		(mol/mol of LDL)
	Mean	±S.D.	Mean
α-Tocopherol	11.58	±3.34	6.37
γ-Tocopherol	0.93	±0.36	0.51
β-Carotene	0.53	±0.47	0.29
α-Carotene	0.22	±0.25	0.12
Lycopene	0.29	±0.20	0.16
Cryptoxanthin	0.25	±0.23	0.14
Cantaxanthin	0.04	±0.07	0.02
Lutein + zeaxanthin	0.07	±0.05	0.04
Ubiquinol-10	0.18	±0.18	0.10

Data taken from [7].

associated with an increased risk of myocardial infarction and coronary artery disease. A possible explanation for the higher atherogenicity of the dense LDL predominant in phenotype B might be that it is more susceptible to oxidation than the less-dense LDL [24,25].

Principles of lipid peroxidation

Oxidation of LDL is a free radical-driven lipid peroxidation process. It starts with the removal of a hydrogen atom, by an initiating radical X·, from one of the polyunsaturated fatty acids (PUFAs) contained in the LDL lipids, according to reaction 1 (note that LH in the reactions is a PUFA bound to one of the LDL lipids). The rate of hydrogen removal (R_i) determines the rate of initiation. This initiation is one of the key steps; however, despite intensive work, the nature of the short-lived primary radical X· is still a mystery, in both most *in vitro* systems (e.g. copper-mediated oxidation) and even more *in vivo*. Once formed, the carbon-centred lipid radical L· reacts very quickly with molecular oxygen, yielding a lipid peroxyl radical, LOO· (reaction 2). The LOO· radical in turn extracts a hydrogen atom from an adjacent lipid, LH, yielding a lipid hydroperoxide, LOOH, and a new lipid radical, L˙ (reaction 3). This reaction is termed chain propagation and proceeds with a given rate constant, k_p.

An interesting feature of such chain reactions is that a single initiating event (reaction 1) could convert a large number of lipids to lipid hydroperoxides. The number of lipid molecules oxidized per initiated radical X˙ depends on several factors, particularly the presence of antioxidants (reaction 4) and the rate of chain termination, when two LOO˙ radicals combine to form non-radical products (reaction 5). If the system contains phenolic antioxidants (AOH), e.g. vitamin E, the LOO˙ radical can be scavenged according to reaction 4, with the consequence that the chain is terminated, because the phenoxyl radical AO˙ has very low reactivity and, under most conditions, does not propagate the lipid peroxidation chain.

Reaction 1: initiation

$$LH + X˙ \xrightarrow{\text{rate} = R_i} L˙ + XH$$

Reaction 2: oxygen addition

$$L˙ + O_2 \xrightarrow{\text{rate, very fast}} LOO˙$$

Reaction 3: chain propagation

$$LOO˙ + LH \xrightarrow{k_p} LOOH + L˙$$

Reaction 4: scavenging by antioxidants

$$LOO˙ + AOH \xrightarrow{k_{inh}} LOOH + AO˙$$

Reaction 5: termination

$$LOO˙ + LOO˙ \xrightarrow{k_t} \text{non-radical product} + O_2$$

In typical experiments the autoxidation is followed by measuring the change in one parameter proportional to the progress of the reaction, i.e. consumption of PUFAs, consumption of oxygen, increase in peroxides or increase in conjugated dienes [26–28]. All methods give equivalent results, but chemists prefer methods which allow continuous monitoring of the progress curves (oxygen uptake, increase in dienes). If the system contains antioxidants, the autoxidation proceeds in two consecutive phases, with quite different rates. Initially, the rate is low, because the antioxidants scavenge LOO˙ radicals (reaction 4) and consequently compete with the propagation. This initial phase is termed lag phase (t_{inh}) or inhibition period. As the reaction proceeds, the antioxidants are consumed and the rate-competing reaction slows down. As a consequence, the rate of propagation accelerates until a maximum rate of uninhibited autoxidation is reached for steady-state conditions. The rate of autoxidation during the lag phase is determined by eqn. 1; the length of the lag phase is directly proportional to the concentration of the antioxidants AOH (eqn. 2), and the maximal rate under uninhibited conditions, when no antioxidants are present, is described by eqn. 3.

$$v_{inh} = \frac{d[LOOH]}{dt} = \frac{k_p[LH]R_i}{n \cdot k_{inh}[AOH]} \tag{1}$$

$$t_{inh} = \text{length of lag phase} = \frac{n[AOH]}{R_i} \tag{2}$$

$$V_{max.} = \frac{d[LOOH]}{dt} = \frac{k_p[LH]R_i^{\frac{1}{2}}}{(2k_t)^{\frac{1}{2}}} \tag{3}$$

In eqn. 2, the factor n is defined as the number of peroxyl radicals (LOO˙) trapped by each molecule of antioxidant. For vitamin E, the value of n is 2, since both vitamin E and the vitamin E radical (tocopheroxyl radical) trap LOO˙. Eqn. 2 also shows that the length of the lag phase is directly proportional to the concentration of the antioxidants, which can scavenge peroxyl radicals, and inversely proportional to the rate, R_i, by which the initiating radicals are formed in reaction 1.

An intrinsic problem in the determination of rate constants in lipid peroxidation is the uncertainty about the rate of initiation, R_i, according to reaction 1, and it is clear that, without knowing R_i, the absolute rate constants cannot be obtained. One possible way of overcoming this problem is to introduce into the reaction mixture a compound which decomposes at a constant rate to free radicals (X˙) capable of extracting a hydrogen atom from the PUFAs according to reaction 1 and consequently initiating the autoxidation process. The compounds most frequently used for this are the so-called azo-initiators (X–N=N–X) which thermally decompose to highly reactive carbon-centred radicals (reaction 6).

Reaction 6: initiation by azo-compounds

$$X—N{=}N—X \xrightarrow{k_d} 2X˙ + N_2$$
$$LH + X˙ \xrightarrow{\text{Rate} = R_i} XH + L˙$$

The water-soluble azo-initiator AAPH [2,2′-azo-bis-(2-amidinopropane) dihydrochloride] can be used to produce radicals in the aqueous phase, whereas the lipid-soluble AMVN [2,2′-azo-bis-(2,4-dimethylvaleronitrile)] can be used to produce radicals in the lipid phase. AAPH decomposes with a first-order rate constant of $k_d = 6.6 \times 10^{-5}/\text{min}$ at 37°C, and the flux of free radicals is directly proportional to the AAPH concentration.

A crucial point is that the rate of initiation (R_i) by AAPH additionally depends on the initiator efficacy (e), i.e. the number of primordial radicals $(X^{.})$ that initiate according to the reaction $R_i = [\text{AAPH}] \times 2 \, kd_e$. Absolute measurement of the initiator efficacy by independent methods is extremely difficult and, therefore, R_i is generally measured indirectly, by the so-called 'induction period method' based on eqn. 2. Briefly, a defined amount of α-tocopherol or the water-soluble analogue trolox is added to the sample to be oxidized. The oxidation is initiated by AAPH and the length of the lag phase, t_{inh}, is measured. The R_i value is then assumed to be $R_i = 2[\alpha\text{-toco-pherol}]/t_{inh}$. In the case of samples containing endogenous vitamin E (e.g. LDL) its initial concentration is used as an internal calibration standard for R_i measurements [28–30].

As mentioned above, AAPH has the advantage that the rate of initiation can be adjusted by variation of the AAPH concentration. For example, a 1 mM AAPH solution gives a rate of initiation (R_i) of about 1.8×10^{-8} M/min if the solution contains LDL in a concentration of 0.5×10^{-6} M, a concentration frequency used in AAPH oxidation studies [28], the rate of initiation per LDL particle is only 0.036 strikes/min, i.e. an LDL particle is hit by a free radical only every 27 min. In a thorough kinetic study, Noguchi et al. [28] have investigated the oxidation of LDL $(0.5 \, \mu\text{M})$ with 1 mM AAPH. The reaction was followed by measuring vitamin E consumption, oxygen uptake, increase of dienes and increase of cholesteryl ester hydroperoxides and phospholipid hydroperoxides. The reaction proceeded in two distinct consecutive phases: an inhibited lag phase during which vitamin E was consumed, and an uninhibited propagation phase. The kinetic chain-length for formation of cholesteryl ester hydroperoxides was 2.9 during the lag phase, and 7.5 during the propagation phase. For formation of phospholipid hydroperoxides, the kinetic chain lengths during the lag and propagation phase were 0.6 and 1.3 respectively. For oxygen consumption, the kinetic chain lengths were 6.3 and 50. This clearly indicates that vitamin E acted as a chain-breaking antioxidant. Similar results were found for oxidation of LDL $(0.5 \, \mu\text{M})$ with $2 \, \mu\text{M}$ copper. These do not support the findings of Bowry and Stocker [31], that the kinetic chain-length in LDL oxidation by AAPH is higher in the presence of vitamin E than in its absence, and that vitamin E acts as a pro-oxidant by chain transfer through the reaction of the tocopheroxyl radical $(\alpha\text{TO}^{.})$ with a lipid molecule, according to the reaction $\alpha\text{TO}^{.} + \text{LH} \rightarrow \alpha\text{TOH} + \text{L}^{.}$.

Kinetics of copper-induced LDL oxidation

Based on many different time-dependent analyses [7], the chronology of LDL oxidation by Cu^{2+} ions can be divided into three consecutive time phases: lag phase, propagation phase and decomposition phase (Fig. 1). During the lag phase, LDL becomes progressively depleted of its antioxidants, with α-toco-

Fig. 1   **Kinetics of copper-stimulated oxidation of LDL, measured by consumption of vitamin E, change in 430 nm fluorescence, lipid hydroperoxides and TBARS**

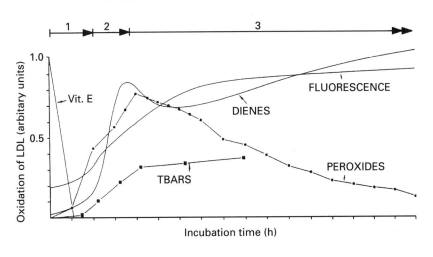

The numbers on top give the length of the lag, propagation and decomposition phase. Abbreviation used: Vit. E, vitamin E.

pherol as the first to leave and β-carotene as the last to remain. During this period, only minimal lipid peroxidation occurs in LDL as seen by the measurement of PUFAs, TBARS (thiobarbituric acid-reactive substances), lipid hydroperoxides, fluorescence and conjugated dienes. Macrophage-mediated LDL oxidation shows the same time sequence. When LDL is depleted of its antioxidants, the rate of lipid peroxidation rapidly accelerates to the maximum rate of the uninhibited process given by eqn. 3. A lipid peroxide peak is reached when about 70–80% of the LDL PUFAs are oxidized, thereafter the peroxide content of LDL starts to decrease again, because decomposition reactions (e.g. formation of aldehydes) become predominant. During the lag and propagation phase, the kinetics of the formation of lipid peroxides, TBARS and fluorescence at 430 nm (excitation 360 nm) closely follow the diene versus time profile, and only after the diene maximum do the different indices separate and follow different kinetics. The second increase of the 234 nm absorption, seen shortly after the peroxide maximum, is not due to newly formed dienes, but to accumulation of decomposition products absorbing at this wavelength.

If PUFAs become oxidized to lipid hydroperoxides, their isolated C=C double bonds are converted to conjugated double bonds showing a strong u.v.-absorption at 234 nm. A convenient and very frequently used method monitoring the process of copper-induced LDL oxidation continuously, is to measure with a spectrophotometer the change of the diene absorption as a function of time as first proposed by our group [32]. An instrument with an automatic cuvette changer allows the measurement of six or more LDL samples simultaneously, which is important for routine analyses. A typical example of such assays is shown in Fig. 2.

Fig. 2   Measurement of oxidation of LDL by the conjugated diene method

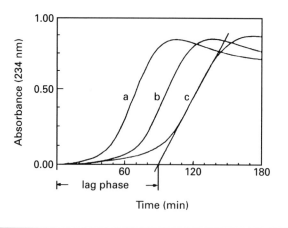

LDL (0.1 μM) isolated from three donors (a, b, c) in phosphate-buffered saline was mixed with 1.66 μM CuCl$_2$ and the change in the 234 nm diene absorption was continuously recorded. The lag phase of LDL from donor C is shown.

The indices which can easily be derived from the diene versus time profiles are the lag phase (t_{inh}, eqn. 2), the maximum rate of oxidation ($V_{max.,}$

eqn. 3) and the maximum amount of dienes produced. If the diene versus time profile is precisely measured, it should also be possible to determine the oxidation rates during the lag phase (eqn. 1) and the rate of peroxide decomposition. Many pitfalls can arise if conditions in copper oxidation are not strictly controlled. The most important factors are: concentration of LDL and Cu^{2+}, ratio of Cu^{2+}/LDL, incubation medium and temperature [33]. Most laboratories using the diene method agree that the method shows excellent reproducibility; for between-runs with the same batch of LDL, the coefficient of variation for t_{inh} and $V_{max.}$ is less than 5% [9,33]. Nevertheless, the mean lag time reported by various laboratories in recent papers for LDL from healthy controls ranges from 68 to 124 min [9]. This wide variation probably reflects minor, but nevertheless important, methodological differences.

The mechanism of how Cu^{2+} induces lipid peroxidation in LDL is still poorly understood. It seems very likely that Cu^{2+} binds to discrete sites of the apo B and forms centres for repeated free radical production similar to those proposed for other biological systems [34]. The number of binding sites in apo B is not exactly known. Values ranging from three to about ten have been reported [7,35]. Any compound which displaces Cu^{2+} from the apo-B-binding site (e.g. EDTA, histidine, certain proteins and many other substances), by forming redox-inactive complexes, should then inhibit or fully prevent LDL oxidation. Such inhibitory effects of Cu^{2+} chelators have been frequently reported [7, 11]. The interaction of medium components with Cu^{2+} explains why lag phases are much longer in F10 medium than in phosphate buffer.

Once bound, Cu^{2+} must be reductively activated by the net transfer of one electron (reaction 7). It is likely that reaction 7 is rate limiting and therefore equal to the rate by which lipid peroxidation is initiated in LDL (reaction 1). The rate of initiation would then also be essential for the length of the lag phase (eqn. 2).

In the case of LDL in phosphate buffer, the required reducing equivalents must be provided either from apo B (e.g. cysteine residues, reaction 7b) or from the lipids (e.g. preformed peroxides, reaction 7c). In the case of oxidation by cells, additional reducing components (e.g. thiols, superoxide anions) released by the cells probably enhance the rate of site-specific reduction of Cu^{2+} and therefore accelerate initiation. An involvement of thiols in transition metal ion-dependent cell-mediated oxidation was first proposed by Heinecke et al. [36]. Sparrow et al. [37] have recently presented evidence that the oxidation of LDL by endothelial cells and macrophages in media containing transition metal ions is caused by the cell-dependent appearance of thiol in the medium.

Reaction 7: reductive activation of Cu^{2+}

(a) $Cu^{2+} + e \xrightarrow{\text{Rate}=R_i} Cu^+$

(b) $Cu^{2+} + RSH \rightarrow Cu^+ + \frac{1}{2}RSSR$

(c) $Cu^{2+} + LOOH \rightarrow Cu^+ + LOO^{\cdot} + H^+$

Cuprous ions (Cu^+) are strong pro-oxidants which probably rapidly form the ultimate initiating radicals by a Fenton-type reaction (reaction 8a, 8b) or by a transition complex with molecular oxygen (reaction 8c).

Reaction 8: initiation of lipid peroxidation by Cu^{2+}

(a) $Cu^+ + LOOH \rightarrow Cu^{2+} + OH^- + LO^{\cdot} \rightarrow$ initiates lipid peroxidation

(b) $Cu^+ + HOOH \rightarrow Cu^{2+} + OH^- + OH^{\cdot} \rightarrow$ initiates lipid peroxidation

(c) $Cu^+ + O_2 \rightarrow [Cu^{2+}-O_2^{-\cdot}] \rightarrow$ initiates lipid peroxidation or release of O_2

The principal difference between AAPH- and Cu^{2+}-induced oxidation is that the former system produces a more or less random attack of free radicals in LDL, whereas the latter involves a site-specific mechanism, which probably has more relevance for the situation *in vivo*. Pro-oxidant copper and iron are present in human atherosclerotic lesions [38]. Moreover, the lag phase in AAPH oxidation is determined in the first place by vitamin E, whereas in copper oxidation the overall lag phase most probably reflects the contribution of all antioxidants, the rate of initiation R_i and perhaps structural parameters of LDL.

Aldehydes

The decomposition of lipid hydroperoxides to aldehydes is a general phenomenon in fat autoxidation and lipid peroxidation in biological systems [39]. These secondary reactions are strongly accelerated by transition metal ions decomposing lipid hydroperoxides to lipid alkoxyl radicals in a Fenton-type reaction, e.g. $LOOH + Fe^{2+} \rightarrow LO^{\cdot} + OH^- + Fe^{3+}$ (see Fig. 3). The lipid alkoxyl radicals undergo β-cleavage reactions (homolytic scission) of the two C–C bonds on either side of the alkoxy group, yielding aldehydes and carbon-centred lipid radicals. If this mechanism is applied to the phospholipid and cholesteryl ester hydroperoxides contained in oLDL, the cleavage of the carbon bonds results in two classes of aldehydes: (i) aliphatic aldehydes derived from the methyl terminus of the fatty acid chain and (ii) aldehyde still bound to the parent lipid molecule, i.e. so-called core aldehydes. The cholesteryl ester core aldehydes are discussed together with the oxysterols (see section entitled Oxysterols).

Fig. 3   Decomposition of lipid hydroperoxides by β-cleavage yields aldehydes

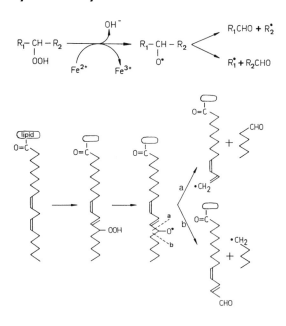

The lower part shows that two classes of aldehydes are formed (a), aldehydes derived from the methylterminus of the fatty acids (hexanal is shown) and (b) core aldehydes bound to the parent lipid molecule.

Phospholipid core aldehydes are almost certainly present in oLDL, but have not yet been investigated. The aliphatic aldehydes found in oLDL are listed in Table 3. The time-course of aldehyde accumulation in LDL oxidized by copper has a lag phase of about 1–2 h with minimal formation of aldehydes followed by a rapid increase lasting about 6 h, thereafter the aldehyde content of LDL remains more or less constant (e.g. 4-hydroxyhexenal) or continues to increase slightly (e.g. malonaldehyde, hexanal, 4-hydroxynonenal). All aldehydes listed in Table 3, except malonaldehyde, are lipophilic compounds and remain largely associated with the LDL particle [40]. On the other hand, malonaldehyde exists at pH 7.4 as the hydrophilic enolate anion ($^-$O–CH=CH–CHO) and about 80–90% diffuses out of the LDL particle into the aqueous phase. It should be noted that what is measured with the TBA-assay (i.e. TBARS) is a good reflection of the level of free malonaldehyde measured by h.p.l.c., suggesting that other oxidized lipids in oLDL interfere to a low extent with the TBA assay.

Table 3   Aldehydes in LDL oxidized with copper for 4–5 h and 20–24 h

	Aldehyde composition (nmol/mg of protein)	
	4–5 h	20–24 h
Hexanal	52	229
Malonaldehyde	86	114
4-Hydroxynonenal	25	114
Nonanal	10	27
4-Hydroxyhexenal	8	49
4-Hydroxyoctenal	7	ND
Propanal	6	ND
Pentanal	5	ND
2,4-Heptadienal	5	ND
Butanal	4	ND
Octanal	1	5
Total aldehydes	209	538

Table compiled from [7]. ND, not determined.

The total amount of free aldehydes, including malonaldehyde, present in LDL after 24 h oxidation is in the range of 540 nmol/mg of protein. This is the largest individual class of products identified so far in oLDL. The distribution (mol %) is: 42% hexanal, 21% malonaldehyde, 21% 4-hydroxynonenal, 9% 4-hydroxyhexenal and 6% other aldehydes. The concentration of hexanal and 4-hydroxynonenal in the LDL lipid phase is extremely high (in the range of 300 and 150 mM respectively). Hexanal and 4-hydroxynonenal arise from oxidation of the ω-6 PUFAs, linoleic acid (18:2) and arachidonic acid (20:4). 4-Hydroxyhexenal and propanal arise from oxidation of the ω-3 PUFA docosahexaenoic acid (22:6). The major, if not the only, source of malonaldehydes are fatty acids with more than three double bonds, i.e. 20:4 and 22:6. Frankel *et al.* [41] recently proposed the determination of hexanal by a rapid headspace gas chromatographic method for assessment of the resistance of LDL to copper oxidation. The amount of hexanal found in oLDL samples (1 mg protein/ml, 8 μM Cu^{2+}, 37°C, 4 h) from different donors correlated ($p < 0.05$, $r = 0.59 - 0.61$) with the PUFA and linoleic acid content of LDL, but no significant correlation was seen with vitamin E. The headspace chromatograms also showed peaks of pentane, propanal and pentanal. Using the hexanal assay, Frankel *et al.* [42] showed that inclusion of certain phenolic antioxidants in the LDL–copper system can inhibit formation of hexanal up to 100%. Red wine phenolics appear to be particularly powerful, a 500- to 1000-fold dilution inhibited hexanal formation by 96% and 100% respectively [42]. H-Proton-n.m.r. spectroscopy of lipid extracts from oLDL showed various signals indicative of aldehydes [43].

Various lines of research [1,7] suggest that important changes occurring in apo B during oxidation result from the reaction of aldehydes with amino acid residues. The strong increase of the 430 nm fluorescence of apo B and the concomitant loss of free amino groups is, for example, probably caused by the reaction of aldehydes with ε-amino groups of lysine residues. Similarly, the strong increase in the net negative surface charge of the LDL particle is attributed to the loss of positively charged amino groups by Schiff's base formation (RCHO + protein $NH_3^+ \rightarrow R–CH=N–protein + H_2O + H^+$) or formation of Michael adducts with α-β-unsaturated aldehydes (R–CH=CH–CHO + protein $NH_3^+ \rightarrow R–CH(NH protein)–CH_2–CHO + H^+$). Uchida *et al.* [44,45] have shown that 4-hydroxynonenal can react with histidine, lysine and cysteine residues in proteins. The products formed are Michael-type adducts in which the carbonyl function is either preserved or has undergone secondary reactions with amino groups to yield inter- and intramolecular cross-links. The complex pattern of reactions given by 4-hydroxynonenal is also evident from a study by Sayre *et al.* [46] suggesting that primary amines condense with the aldehyde to form pyrrole derivatives under physiological conditions.

Antibodies prepared against malonaldehyde and 4-hydroxynonenal-treated native LDL also react with copper- or cell-oLDL, indicating that these aldehyde conjugates are indeed epitopes of apo B newly formed during oxidation [7]. More importantly, immunohistochemical methods have clearly shown that malonaldehyde- and 4-hydroxynonenal-modified apo B occurs in atherosclerotic lesions of rabbits [47] and humans [48]. In human aorta the thickened intima of initial, transitional and advanced lesions and atheromata showed predominantly extracellular staining with antibodies specific for 4-hydroxynonenal-epitopes [48]. Moreover, auto-antibodies directed against malonaldehyde- or 4-hydroxynonenal-modified proteins are present in the serum of rabbits and humans [7]. The titre of auto-antibodies to malonaldehyde-modified LDL was highly significantly correlated with the progression of human carotid atherosclerosis [49].

Many of the chemical (e.g. loss of NH_2-groups), physicochemical (e.g. increase of fluorescence and electrophoretic mobility) and biological (e.g macrophage uptake, cytotoxicity) properties of cell- or copper-oxidized LDL can be reproduced in full or in part by the treatment of previously non-oxidized LDL with aldehydes or aldehyde mixtures [1,7,50–53]. Aminoguanidine, a compound presently in clinical trials for inhibiting formation of advanced glycosylation products in chronic hyperglycaemia, inhibits the oxidative modification of LDL *in vitro*, presumably by binding reactive aldehydes and preventing their conjugation to apo B [54]. The precise chemical structure of the aldehyde apo B conjugates and their location on the apo B polypeptide chain remain to be determined. Fruebis *et al.* [55] examined the interaction of phospholipid hydroperoxides with peptides and proposed that, in the first step, adducts between lipid radicals and protein amino groups are formed, which in a second oxidation step form protein-linked aldehydes.

Hydroperoxy and hydroxy fatty acids

The change in the lipid and fatty acid composition of LDL caused by copper oxidation is shown in Table 4. The amount of total hydroperoxides formed in LDL during copper oxidation in phosphate-buffered saline (PBS) was measured iodometrically by a simple commercial assay [7,32,56]. After a certain lag period of 1–2 h, total peroxides rapidly increased and reached a maximum of about 700–1000 nmol peroxides/mg of LDL protein after 4–5 h. Thereafter, total peroxides decreased again and were hardly detectable 24 h after initiation of oxidation (Table 5). Using a similar peroxide assay, Jessup *et al.* [57] found the same time-course for total peroxides in oxidation of LDL by mouse peritoneal macrophages in Ham's F10 supplemented with $3 \mu M$ FeSO$_4$, and in cell-free Ham's F10 medium supplemented with $100 \mu M$ Cu^{2+}. Stocker *et al.* [19] were among the first who employed a newly developed h.p.l.c. method, which allows the separation and detection of cholesteryl ester hydroperoxides, phospholipid hydroperoxides and triglyceride hydroperoxides in a highly sensitive and selective manner. LDL oxidized with 1 mM AAPH for 3 h contained substantial amounts of all three hydroperoxide classes with a molar ratio of about 5:2:1. This group did not investigate copper-oxidized LDL, but they reported that LDL exposed to activated polymorphonuclear neutrophils for 2 h also contained significantly increased levels of cholesteryl ester hydroperoxides, phospholipid hydroperoxides and triglyceride hydroperoxides. Noguchi *et al.* [28] measured the time-course of the formation of total phospholipid hydroperoxides and total cholesteryl ester hydroperoxides with h.p.l.c. and detection at 234 nm (this wavelength is not specific for hydroperoxides, but for conjugated dienes, which could include both hydroperoxides and the corresponding reduced monohydroxy compound). It was found that in LDL (0.25 mg protein/ml) exposed to copper ($2 \mu M$), cholesteryl ester hydroperoxides and phospholipid hydroper-oxides rise slowly during the first 2 h, then the increase occurs more rapidly to a level of about $45 \mu M$ (= 180 nmol cholesteryl ester hydroperoxides/mg of protein) and $15 \mu M$ (= 60 mg phospholipid hydroperoxide/mg of protein) (Table 5). After 5 h the cholesteryl ester hydroperoxides tended to decrease, whereas phospholipid hydroperoxides still increased. The cholesteryl ester and phospholipid hydroper-oxide contents in LDL oxidized for 5 h with AAPH (1 mM) were approximately

Table 4   Change of lipid, fatty acid and antioxidant
composition of LDL caused by copper oxidation

	Change observed	References
Phosphatidylcholine	Decrease to 65–55%	[60,61]
Lysophosphatidylcholine	Strong increase to approx 400 nmol/mg of protein	[60,61]
Sphingomyelin	Not studied	
Triglycerides	Decrease to 76–52%	[60–62]
Free cholesterol	Decrease to 90–50%	[60,61-64]
Cholesteryl ester	Decrease to 48–25%	[62,64]
Total cholesterol	Decrease to 78–30%	[60–63]
Palmitic acid	No change	[7]
Stearic acid	Decrease to 96–79%	[7,59]
Oleic acid	Decrease to 80–46%	[7,59]
Linoleic acid	Decrease to 15–0%	[7,58,59]
Arachidonic acid	Complete consumption	[7,58,59]
Docosahexaenoic acid	Complete consumption	[7]
Vitamin E	Complete consumption	[7]
Carotenoids	Complete consumption	[7]

Data were taken from the following references:
[60] 0.2–0.4 μM LDL, 5 μM Cu²⁺ in phosphate-buffered saline (PBS), 37°C, 24 h;
[61] 0.4 μM LDL, 5 μM Cu²⁺ in PBS, 37°C, 29 h;
[62] 0.4 μM LDL, 25 μM Cu²⁺ in PBS, 4°C, 48 h;
[7] 0.2–0.4 μM LDL, 3–6 μM Cu²⁺ in PBS, ambient temp., 24 h;
[59] 0.4 μM LDL, 20 μM Cu²⁺ in Ham's F10, 37°C, 1.5 and 20 h;
[58] 30 μM LDL, 5 μM Cu²⁺, ambient temp., 24 h;
[63] 0.4 μM LDL, 20 μM Cu²⁺ in PBS, 24 h;
[64] 0.4 μM LDL, 5 μM Cu²⁺ in PBS, 37°C, 20 h.

120 nmol/mg of protein and 33 nmol/mg of protein respectively. AMVN gave mainly cholesteryl ester hydroperoxides (about 60 nmol/mg of protein), with only trace amounts of phospholipid hydroperoxides. Both phospholipid hydroperoxides and cholesteryl ester hydroperoxides are still a complex mixture of hydroperoxides differing in type of fatty acids (18:2, 20:4, 22:6) and position of the hydroperoxy group [e.g. 9-HODE (9-hydroxy-10,12-octadecadienoic acid) or 13-HODE (13-hydroxy-9,11-octa-decadienoic acid)]. So far, no methodology has been developed which would allow further separation and quantification of the individual species present in the pool of phospholipid or cholesteryl ester peroxides. Investigators interested in more detailed analyses reduce the hydro-

Table 5   Lipid oxidation products demonstrated in copper-oxidized LDL

	Lipid oxidation products (nmol/mg of protein)		
	4–5 h	20–24 h	Reference
Total peroxides	1000	227	[7]
Phospholipid hydroperoxides	60	—	[28]
Cholesteryl ester hydro-peroxides	180	—	[28]
Conjugated dienes	240	—	[28]
TBARS	85	114	[7]
Total aldehydes + TBARS	210	540	[7]
Hydroxyoctadecenoic acid*	7	50	[59]
Hydroxyoctadecadienoic acid†	110	30	[59]
Hydroxyeicosatetraenoic acid‡	17	0	[59]
7-Hydroxy- and 7-hydro-peroxycholesterol	60	120	[63,64]
7-Ketocholesterol	ND	ND	[63–65]
Cholesteroloxoalkanoylester	ND	30	[67]
7-Ketocholesterolalkanoylester	ND	30	[67]
5,6-Epoxycholesterol	ND	Traces	[64,65]
25-Hydroxycholesterol	ND	Traces	[65]
Cholest-3,5-dien-7-one	ND	ND	[63,65]

Data are approximate figures from the various investigations indicated below:
[7] 0.1 μM LDL, 1.66 μM Cu^{2+} in PBS, ambient temp.;
[28] 0.5 μM LDL, 2 μM Cu^{2+} in PBS, 37°C;
[59] 0.4 μM LDL, 20 μM Cu^{2+} in Ham's F10, 37°;
[63] 0.4 μM LDL, 20 μM Cu^{2+} in PBS, 37°C;
[64] 0.4 μM LDL, 5 μM Cu^{2+} in PBS, 37°C;
[65] 0.2–0.4 μM LDL, ? μM Cu^{2+} in M199;
[66] 30 μM LDL, 5 μM Cu^{2+}, ambient temp.

* Sum of 8-, 10- and 11-hydroxy-derivatives of oleic acid.
† Sum of 9-HODE and 13-HODE.
‡ Sum of 5-HETE, 8-HETE, 9-HETE, 11-HETE, 12-HETE and 15-HETE.
ND, not determined.

peroxides present in the bulk LDL lipid extract to the corresponding alcohols, saponify the lipids and separate the monohydroxy fatty acids by gas chromatography. This does not of course allow conclusions regarding the parent lipid molecule to which the hydroperoxy fatty acid was bound. The first study in this area was reported by Lenz et al. [58]. In LDL (1.5 mg protein/ml) oxidized with 5 μM CuSO$_4$ for 24 h they found *trans, cis* and *trans, trans* 13-HODE (92 nmol/mg of protein) and *trans, cis* and *trans, trans* 9-HODE (86 nmol/mg of protein) and the hydroxy fatty acids derived from arachidonic acid, i.e. 5-hydroxy-6,8,11,14-eicosatetraenoic acid (5-HETE; 4.3 nmol), 8-hydroxy-5,9,11,14-eicosatetraenoic acid and 9-hydroxy-5,7,11,14-eicosatetraenoic acid (8-HETE + 9-HETE; 5.9 nmol), 12-hydroxy-5,8,10,14-eicosatetraenoic acid (12-HETE; 4.5 nmol) and 15-hydroxy-5,8,11,13-eicosatetraenoic acid (15-HETE; 4.1 nmol). The time-course showed no increase of HODE and HETE during the first 4 h of incubation. Thereafter, the increase was more or less linear with time up to 24 h. The hydroxy fatty acids accounted for approximately 70% of the linoleate consumed during LDL oxidation and represented 45-fold more products than were measured with the TBARS analyses. It should be noted that in this study [58] a strong variation between the four LDL samples investigated was observed. For example, in one LDL sample most of the linoleic acid and arachidonic acid were still present after 24 h. This is not in agreement with other studies [7,59], which found that linoleic acid and arachidonic acid are more or less completely consumed after 24 h copper oxidation.

In a recent careful study, Wang et al. [59] studied, by g.c./m.s., the time-course of the formation of monohydroxy derivatives of arachidonic acid, linoleic acid and oleic acid during oxidation of LDL (0.2 mg of protein/ml) by 20 μM copper and by endothelial cells. Oxidation of LDL by copper (Table 5) resulted, after a lag phase of about 1 h, in a strong increase of the linoleic acid oxidation products (9-HODE, 13-HODE) and the arachidonic acid oxidation products (5-, 8-, 9-, 11-, 12- and 15-HETE [11-HETE is 11-hydroxy-5,8,12,14-eicosatetraenoic acid]). Interestingly, considerable amounts of the oxidation products of oleic acid (8-, 10- and 11-hydroxyoctadecenoic acid) were also found. The HETEs and HODEs reached a maximum at 5 h and decreased to almost zero after 20 h, whereas the hydroxy derivatives of oleic acid increased up to 24 h. The quantities measured at 5 h oxidation were 110 nmol HETE/mg of protein, 17 nmol HODE/mg of protein, and, after 20 h, 50 nmol hydroxy derivatives of oleic acid. TBAR values after 20 h reached 60 nmol/mg of protein. In this study it was also demonstrated that 99% of the hydroxy fatty acids remain associated with the LDL particle, as evident by re-isolation of the oLDL by ultracentrifugation. Oxidation of LDL by endothelial cells gave a similar product pattern to oxidation by copper ions and there was little positional specificity, suggesting that in endothelial cell oxidation as well the majority of the fatty acid oxidation products are formed via non-enzymic lipid peroxidation processes.

Oxysterols

Oxidation of LDL lipids is not restricted to the PUFAs; a number of more recent studies demonstrated that the cholesterol moiety can also be oxygenated. Zhang *et al.* [64] reported that Cu^{2+}–oxidized LDL contains 7-ketocholesterol, 7-hydroxycholesterol and 5,6-epoxycholesterol, with 7-ketocholesterol constituting the abundant sterol oxidation products. Unlike Zhang *et al.* [64], Bhadra *et al.* [65] found cholest-3,5-dien-7-one as the major product in Cu^{2+}-oxidized LDL, with smaller amounts of 5,6-epoxycholesterol, 7-hydroxycholesterol, 7-ketocholesterol and 25-hydroxy cholesterol. Endothelial cell-oxidized LDL contained only the 5,6-epoxycholesterol [65]. Malavasi *et al.* [63] followed the time-course of cholesterol oxidation (0.2 mg protein/ml) with $20\,\mu M$ $CuSO_4$ in PBS at 37°C, and found that 7-hydroperoxy cholesterol ($7\alpha OOH$, $7\beta OOH$) is largely prevalent at early stages of oxidation. The concentration of the hydroperoxides decreases with oxidation time, with concomitant formation of 7-hydroxycholesterol ($7\alpha OH$, $7\beta OH$) and cholest-3,5-dien-7-one. The total amount of oxysterols increased during the first 12 h from zero to about $50\,\mu g/mg$ of protein, and then started to decrease again. After 24 h, about 54% of the total LDL cholesterol was consumed. Incubation of plasma with copper ions (0.5–2 mM, 24 h, 37°C) gives rise to the formation of free and esterified oxysterols, mainly 7-ketocholesterol, 7-hydroxycholesterol and 5,6-epoxycholesterol [66]. Esterbauer *et al.* [7,11,39] have repeatedly proposed that the oxidation of phospholipids or cholesteryl ester yields, in addition to the aldehyde fragments derived from the methyl terminus of fatty acid chains, the counterpart aldehydes, where the fragmented fatty acid chains are still bound to the parent lipid molecules (Fig. 3). Kamido *et al.* [67] first demonstrated that lipid peroxidation of cholesteryl esters and phospholipids leads to formation of cholesteryl oxoalkanoates and phospholipid oxoalkanoates. To this new class of lipid-derived aldehydes was given the name 'core aldehyde'. About 1–2% of the cholesteryl linoleate and cholesteryl arachidonate consumed upon copper oxidation of LDL are core aldehydes. 7-Cholesteryl ester core aldehydes and 7-ketocholesteryl ester core aldehydes were identified. In both series the aldehydes had chain lengths of between four and 10 carbon atoms. The C_9 core aldehydes (cholesteryl-9-oxo-nonanoate and 7-ketocholesterol-9-oxo-nonanoate) comprised about 60% of the main core aldehydes, followed by the C_8 core aldehydes ($\approx 20\%$) and C_5 core aldehydes (8–10%). The parent lipids are most probably cholesteryl linoleate for the C_9 aldehydes and cholesteryl arachidonate for the C_5 aldehydes. The C_8 aldehydes might arise from traces of cholesteryl eicosatrienoic acid (*n*-6) or double bond migration during peroxidation.

It can be seen that the identification and quantification of oxysterols and cholesteryl ester core aldehydes is still at an early stage. Since some of these products are biologically very active this subject deserves further attention. For example, Carpenter *et al.* [68] have shown that cultured human monocyte-macrophages oxidize a cholesteryl linoleate–albumin complex to 7-hydroxycholesterol and 9- and 13-HODE. In lipids extracted from atheroma, 26-hydroxycholesterol, 7-hydroxycholesterol and isomeric HODEs were detected [69]. Hodis *et al.* [70] reported that probucol reduces plasma and aortic wall oxysterol levels (7-hydroxycholesterol, 5,6-epoxycholesterol and 3,5,6-cholestanetriol) in cholesterol-fed rabbits. A similar observation was also made in probucol-treated Watanabe heritable hyperlipidaemic rabbits [71], where a significant reduction in plasma levels of 7α-hydroxycholesterol, 3,5,6-cholestanetriol, 7-ketocholesterol and 25-hydroxycholesterol was found. Rabbits treated with butylated hydroxytoluene showed decreased plasma levels of 7-ketocholesterol and 5,6-epoxycholesterol [72]. Cholestanetriols (e.g. 3β, 5α, 6β) and 25-hydroxycholesterol have been shown to cause injury to endothelial cells and smooth muscle cells, and to alter LDL receptor functions [73].

Some oxysterols (7-hydroxycholesterol, 3,7,22-cholestanetriol, 3,5,6-cholestanetriol and 5,6-epoxycholesterol) are highly toxic for endothelial cells at concentrations in the range of 15–50 nmol/ml [74,75]. Zwijsen *et al.* [76] have shown that oxysterols inhibit gap junctional intercellular communications of smooth muscle cells by more than 40% at concentrations of 1–10 nmol/ml. The inhibitory activity increased in the order: 5,6-epoxycholesterol < 7-ketocholesterol < 3,5,6-cholestanetriol < 25-hydroxycholesterol. A disturbance of intercellular communication may result in disturbances of growth and induction of proliferation of smooth muscle cells.

Lipoxygenase oxidation of LDL

The first study on lipoxygenase-mediated LDL oxidation was reported by Sparrow *et al.* [77], who showed that soybean lipoxygenase, a plant derived 15-lipoxygenase, in combination with phospholipase A_2 is capable of converting LDL into a form with increased TBARS, relative electrophoretic mobility and macrophage uptake. Cathcart *et al.* [78] showed that soybean lipoxygenase can also oxidize LDL in the absence of phospholipase A_2, as evident by dienes, TBARS and cytotoxicity. Several attempts were later made to demonstrate whether lipoxygenases are involved in cell-mediated oxidation of LDL. Lipoxygenase inhibitors indeed blocked modification of LDL by rabbit endothelial cells [79], human monocytes [80] and mouse peritoneal macrophages [81]. However, the high concentration of inhibitors required, and their rather non-specific character, made the involvement of lipoxygenases in cell-mediated oxidation questionable. In several studies, it was clearly demonstrated that 5-lipoxygenases are not responsible for oxidation of LDL by mouse peritoneal macrophages [82,83] and human monocytes [84]. On the other hand, it was shown that 15-lipoxygenases occur in human and rabbit atherosclerotic lesions and are co-localized with deposits of oLDL [85,86]. Belkner *et al.* [87] studied the oxygenation of LDL by purified rabbit reticulocyte 15-lipoxygenase and recombinant human 15-lipoxygenase. This enzyme converts free arachidonic acid and linoleic acid into the 15-hydroperoxy eicosatetraenoic acid and 13-hydroperoxy-octadecadienoic acid. The enzyme can also convert arachidonic acid and linoleic acid bound to phospholipids and cholesteryl ester to the corresponding 15- and 13-hydroperoxy lipids. Incubation of LDL with 15-lipoxygenase at a molar ratio of 17:1 (molecular mass of lipoxygenase = 75 kDa) leads to the oxidation of about 0.5% of the linoleic acid residues in LDL within 30 min. This corresponds to a turnover of approx. three linoleate molecules/min produced by one lipoxygenase molecule. Analyses of the oxygenated polyenic fatty acids (after reduction and alkaline hydrolysis) revealed 13-hydroxy-9-*cis*, 11-*trans*-octadecadienoic acid (13-HODE, Z,E) as the main product (71%), with lower amounts of 15-HETE (10%), 13-hydroxy-9-*trans*, 11-*trans*-octadecadienoic acid (5%) and 9-HODE (17%). At low LDL concentrations, the *S*-isomer of 13-HODE and 15-HETE was formed predominantly. More than 90% of the hydroxy fatty acids were contained in the esterified lipid fraction, particularly in the cholesteryl esters. Long-time treatment (20 h) or high concentrations of lipoxygenase also altered the apo B, as demonstrated by the increased electrophoretic mobility and the increased content of Schiff's bases in apo B. This suggests that a fraction of the hydroperoxides decompose, probably catalysed by traces of transition metal ions present in the incubation mixture. It is important to mention that also in the lipoxygenase-mediated oxidation, oxygen uptake is about two-fold higher than formation of hydroxy fatty acids. A similar observation was made in AAPH- or copper-induced LDL oxidation [28]. The fate of this additionally consumed oxygen and where it is bound is not clear.

In human plasma incubated with reticulocyte 15-lipoxygenase, 13-HODE (main product), 9-HODE and 15-HETE esterified with cholesterol were formed [88]. Moreover, lipids extracted from pieces of atherotic aortas of patients who died from acute heart failure contain considerable amounts of cholesterol esterified with keto- and hydroxyoctadecadienoic acid [89]. The non-specific product pattern of the arterial wall material regarding positional and stereoisomers suggest that, *in vivo*, non-enzymic peroxidation processes are responsible for formation of the majority of these oxygenated fatty acids. Of course, cellular 15-lipoxygenase of endothelial cells or monocyte-macrophages could play an important role for the initiation of the non-enzymic lipid peroxidation process, by providing seed-hydroperoxides in LDL. Even small amounts of peroxides would render LDL susceptible to a subsequent non-enzymic oxidation mediated by free or complexed transition metal ions.

Oxidation of LDL with human umbilical vein endothelial cells in Ham's F10 medium for 20 h also yielded an oxygenated fatty acid pattern characteristic of a non-enzymic peroxidation [59]. The main products identified were the monohydroxy derivatives of linoleic acid (9-HODE, 13-HODE) and arachidonic acid (5-HETE, 8-HETE, 9-HETE, 11-HETE, 12-HETE, 15-HETE). Small amounts of hydroxylated derivatives of oleic acid (8-hydroxy, 10-hydroxy and 11-hydroxy; 18:1) were also formed. The total amount of monohydroxy fatty acids was about 22 nmol/mg of LDL protein (= 12 mol/mol of LDL) with 54% HODEs and 45% HETEs. The isomer distribution in LDL oxidized for 5 h with Cu^{2+} was identical to that in endothelial cell-oxidized LDL. The total amount of monohydroxy fatty acids in Cu^{2+}-oxidized LDL, however, was around 150 nmol/mg of LDL protein.

The authors gratefully acknowledges that Portland Press has given permission for a modified and updated version of this article to be published in Rev. Physiol. Biochem. Pharmacol. The author's work has been supported by the Association for International Cancer Research (AICR), UK, and by the Jubiläumsfonds der Österreichischen Nationalbank, Project No. 4484.

References

1. Juergens, G., Hoff, H.F., Chisolm, G.M. and Esterbauer, H. (1987) Chem. Phys. Lipids **45**, 315–336
2. Steinberg, D., Parthasarathy, S., Carew, T.E., Khoo, J.C. and Witztum, J.L. (1989) N. Engl. J. Med. **320**, 915–924
3. Steinbrecher, U.P., Zhang, H. and Lougheed, M. (1990) Free Radical Biol. Med. **9**, 155–168
4. Bruckdorfer, K.R. (1990) Curr. Opin. Lipidol. **1**, 529–535
5. Lyons, T.J. (1991) Diabetic Med. **8**, 411–419
6. Carpenter, K.L.H., Brabbs, C.E. and Mitchinson, M.J. (1991) Klin. Wochenschr. **69**, 1039–1045
7. Esterbauer, H., Gebicki, J., Puhl, H. and Juergens, G. (1992) Free Radical Biol. Med. **13**, 341–390
8. Leake, D.S. (1993) Br. Heart J. **69**, 476–478
9. Esterbauer, H. and Juergens, G. (1993) Curr. Opin. Lipidol. **4**, 114–124
10. Halliwell, B. (1993) Haemostasis **23** (Suppl. 1), 118–126
11. Gebicki, J., Juergens, G. and Esterbauer, H. (1991) in Oxidative Stress (Sies, H., ed.), pp. 371–397, Academic Press, London
12. Haberland, M.E. and Steinbrecher, U.P. (1992) in Molecular Genetics of Coronary Artery Disease: Candidate Genes and Processes in Atherosclerosis (Lusis, A.J., Rotter, J.I. and Sparkes, R.S., eds.), pp. 35–61, Karger, Basel
13. Chisolm, G.M. (1992) in Biological Consequences of Oxidative Stress: Implications for Cardiovascular Disease and Carcinogenesis (Spatz, L. and Bloom, A.D., eds.), pp. 78–106, Oxford University Press, Oxford
14. Frostegard, J., Wu, R., Giscombe, R., Holm, G., Lefvert, A.K. and Nilsson, J. (1992) Arterioscler. Thromb. **12**, 461–467
15. Zwijsen, R.M.L., Japenga, S.C., Heijen, A.M.P., Van den Bos, R.C. and Koeman, J.H. (1992) Biochem. Biophys. Res. Commun. **186**, 1410–1416
16. Jougasaki, M., Kugiyama, K., Saito, Y., Nakao, K., Imura, H. and Yasue, H. (1992) Circ. Res. **71**, 614–619
17. Sommer, A., Prenner, E., Gorges, R., StÅtz, H., Grillhofer, H., Kostner, G.M., Paltauf, F. and Hermetter, A. (1992) J. Biol. Chem. **267**, 24217–24222
18. Vance, J.E. (1990) Biochim. Biophys. Acta **1045**, 128–134
19. Stocker, R., Bowry, V.W. and Frei, B. (1991) Proc. Natl. Acad. Sci. U.S.A. **38**, 1646–1650
20. Mohr, D., Bowry, V.W. and Stocker, R. (1992) Biochim. Biophys. Acta **1126**, 247–254
21. Yang, C. and Pownall, H.J. (1993) in Structure and Function of Apolipoproteins (Rosseneu, M., ed.), pp. 64–84, CRC Press, Boca Raton
22. Camejo, G., Lopez, A., Lopez, F. and Quinones, J. (1985) Atherosclerosis **55**, 93

23. Campos, H., Blijlevens, E., McNamara, J.R., Ordovas, J.M., Posner, B.M., Wilson, P.W.F., Castelli, W.P. and Schaffer, E.J. (1992) Arterioscler. Thromb. **12**, 1410–1419

24. De Graaf, J., Hak-Lemmers, H.L.M., Hectors, M.P.C., Demacker, P.N.M., Hendricks, J.C.M. and Stalenhoef, A.F.H. (1991) Arterioscler. Thromb. **11**, 298–306

25. Tribble, D.L., Holl, L.G., Wood, P.D. and Krauss, R.M. (1992) Atherosclerosis **93**, 189–199

26. Cosgrove, J.P., Church, D.F. and Pryor, W.A. (1987) Lipids **22**, 299–304

27. Niki, E. (1987) Br. J. Cancer **55**, 153–157

28. Noguchi, N., Gotoh, N. and Niki, E. (1993) Biochim. Biophys. Acta **1168**, 348–357

29. Sato, K., Niki, E. and Shimasaki, H. (1990) Arch. Biochem. Biophys. **279**, 402–405

30. Mino, M., Miki, M., Miyake, M. and Ogiahara, T. (1989) Ann. N.Y. Acad. Sci. **570**, 296–310

31. Bowry, V.W. and Stocker, R. (1993) J. Am. Chem. Soc. **115**, 6029–6044

32. Esterbauer, H., Striegl, G., Puhl, H. and Rotheneder, M. (1989) Free Radical Res. Commun. **6**, 67–75

33. Kleinveld, H.A., Hak-Lemmers, H.L.M., Stalenhoef, A.F.H. and Demacker, P.N.M. (1992) Clin. Chem. **38**, 2066–2072

34. Chevion, M. (1988) Free Radical Biol. Med. **5**, 27–37

35. Kuzuya, M., Yamada, K., Hayashi, T., Funaki, C., Naito, M., Asai, K. and Cuzuya, F. (1992) Biochim. Biophys. Acta **1123**, 334–341

36. Heinecke, J.W., Rosen, H., Suzuki, L.A. and Chait, A. (1987) J. Biol. Chem. **262**, 10098–10103

37. Sparrow, C.P. and Olszewski, J. (1993) J. Lipid Res. **34**, 1219–1228

38. Smith, C., Mitchinson, M.J., Aruoma, O.I. and Halliwell, B. (1992) Biochem. J. **286**, 901–905

39. Esterbauer, H., Zollner, H. and Schaur, R. (1990) in Membrane Lipid Oxidation (Pelfrey, C., ed.), pp. 239–268, CRC Press, Boca Raton

40. Esterbauer, H., Juergens, G., Quehenberger, O. and Koller, E. (1987) J. Lipid Res. **28**, 495–509

41. Frankel, E.N., German, J.B. and Davis, P.A. (1992) Lipids **27**, 1047–1051

42. Frankel, E.N., Kanner, J., German, J.B., Parks, E. and Kinsella, J.E. (1993) Lancet **341**, 454–457

43. Lodge, J.K., Patel, S.U. and Sadler, P.J. (1993) Biochem. J. **289**, 149–153

44. Uchida, K. and Stadtman, E.R. (1992) Proc. Natl. Acad. Sci. U.S.A. **89**, 4544–4548

45. Uchida, K. and Stadtman, E.R. (1993) J. Biol. Chem. **268**, 6388–6393

46. Sayre, L.M., Arora, P.K., Iyer, R.S. and Salomon, R.G. (1993) Chem. Res. Toxicol. **6**, 19–22

47. Palinski, W., Ylä-Herttuala, S., Rosenfeld, M.E., Butler, S.W., Socher, S.A., Parthasarathy, S., Curtiss, L.K. and Witztum, J.L. (1990) Arteriosclerosis **10**, 325–335

48. Juergens, G., Chen, Q., Esterbauer, H., Mair, S., Ledinski, G. and Dinges, H.P. (1993) Arterioscler. Thromb., **13**, 1689–1699

49. Salonen, J., Ylä-Herttuala, S., Yamamoto, R., Butler, S., Korpela, H., Salonen, R, Nyyssînen, K., Palinski, W. and Witztum, J.L. (1992) Lancet **339**, 883–887

50. Hoff, H.F., O'Neill, J., Chisolm, G.M., Cole, T.B., Quehenberger, O., Esterbauer, H. and Juergens, G. (1989) Arteriosclerosis **9**, 538–549

51. Hoff, H.F. and Cole, T.B. (1991) Lab. Invest. **64**, 254–264

52. Hoff, H.F. and O'Neil, J. (1993) J. Lipid Res. **34**, 1209–1217

53. Jessup, W., Juergens, G., Lang, J., Esterbauer, H. and Dean, R.T. (1986) Biochem. J. **234**, 245–248

54. Picard, S., Parthasarathy, S., Fruebis, J. and Witztum, J.L. (1992) Proc. Natl. Acad. Sci. U.S.A. **89**, 6876–6880

55. Fruebis, J., Parthasarathy, S. and Steinberg, D. (1992) Proc. Natl. Acad. Sci. U.S.A. **89**, 10588–10592

56. El-Saadani, M., Esterbauer, H., El-Sayed, M., Goher, M., Nasser, A.Y. and Juergens, G. (1989) J. Lipid Res. **30**, 627–630

57. Jessup, W., Rankin, S.M., De Whalley, C.V., Hoult, J.R.S., Scott, J. and Leake, D.S. (1990) Biochem. J. **265**, 399–405

58. Lenz, M.L., Hughes, H., Mitchell, J.R., Via, D.P., Guyton, J.R., Taylor, A.A., Gotto, A.M. and Smith, Ch. (1990) J. Lipid Res. **31**, 1043–1050

59. Wang, T., Yu, W. and Powell, W.S. (1992) J. Lipid Res. **33**, 525–537

60. Steinbrecher, U.P., Witztum, J.L., Parthasarathy, S. and Steinberg, D. (1987) Arteriosclerosis 7, 135–143
61. Barenghi, L., Bradamante, S., Giudici, G.A. and Vergani, C. (1990) Free Radical Res. Commun. 8, 175–183
62. Van Hinsbergh, V.W.M., van Scheffer, M., Havekes, L. and Kempen, H.J.M. (1986) Biochim. Biophys. Acta 878, 49–64
63. Malavasi, B., Rasetti, M.F., Roma, P., Fogliatto, R., Allevi, P., Catapano, A.L. and Galli, G. (1992) Chem. Phys. Lipids 62, 209–214
64. Zhang, H., Basra, H.J.K. and Steinbrecher, U.P. (1990) J. Lipid Res. 31, 1361–1369
65. Bhadra, S., Arshad, M.A.Q., Rymaszewski, Z., Norman, E., Wherley, R. and Subbiah, M.T.R. (1991) Biochem. Biophys. Res. Commun. 176, 431–440
66. Tamasawa, N. and Takebe, K. (1992) Tohoku J. Exp. Med. 168, 37–45
67. Kamido, H., Kuksis, A., Marai, L. and Myher, J.J. (1992) FEBS Lett. 304, 269–272
68. Carpenter, K.L.H., Ballantine, J.A., Fussell, B., Enright, J.H. and Mitchinson, M.J. (1990) Atherosclerosis 83, 217–229
69. Carpenter, K.L.H., Taylor, S.E., Ballantine, J.A., Fussell, B., Halliwell, B. and Mitchinson, M.J. (1993) Biochim. Biophys. Acta 1167, 121–130
70. Hodis, H.N., Chauhan, A., Hashimoto, S., Crawford, D.W. and Sevanian, A. (1992) Atherosclerosis 96, 125–134
71. Stalenhoef, A.F.H., Kleinveld, H.A., Kosmeijer-Schuil, T.G., Demacker, P.N.M. and Katan, M.B. (1993) Atherosclerosis 98, 113–114
72. Björkhem, I., Henriksson-Freyschuss, A., Breuer, O., Diczfalusy, U., Berglund, L. and Henriksson, P. (1991) Arterioscler. Thromb. 11, 15–22
73. Peng, S., Hu, B. and Morin, R.J. (1991) J. Clin. Lab. Anal. 5, 144–152
74. Sevanian, A., Berliner, J. and Petterson, H. (1991) J. Lipid Res. 32, 147–155
75. Petterson, K.S., Boberg, K.M., Stabursvik, A. and Prydz, H. (1991) Arterioscler. Thromb. 11, 423–428
76. Zwijsen, R.M.L., Oudenhoven, I.M.J. and de Haan, L.H.J. (1992) Eur. J. Pharmacol. 228, 115–120
77. Sparrow, C.P., Parthasarathy, S. and Steinberg, D. (1988) J. Lipid Res. 29, 745–753
78. Cathcart, M.K., McNally, A.K. and Chisolm, G.M. (1991) J. Lipid Res. 32, 63–70
79. Parthasarathy, S., Wieland, E. and Steinberg, D. (1989) Proc. Natl. Acad. Sci. U.S.A. 86, 1046–1050
80. McNally, A.M., Chisolm, G.M., Morel, D.W. and Cathcart, M.K. (1990) J. Immunol. 145, 254–259
81. Rankin, S.M., Parthasarathy, S. and Steinberg, D. (1991) J. Lipid Res. 32, 449–456
82. Jessup, W., Darley-Usmar, V., O'Leary, V. and Bedwell, S. (1991) Biochem. J. 278, 163–169
83. Sparrow, C.P. and Olszewski, J. (1992) Proc. Natl. Acad. Sci U.S.A. 89, 128–131
84. Folcik, V.A. and Cathcart, M.K. (1993) J. Lipid Res. 34, 69–79
85. Ylä-Herttuala, S., Rosenfeld, M.E., Parthasarathy, S., Glass, C.K., Sigal, E., Witztum, J.L. and Steinberg, D. (1990) Proc. Natl. Acad. Sci. U.S.A. 87, 6959–6963
86. Ylä-Herttuala, S., Rosenfeld, M.E., Parthasarathy, S., Glass, C.K., Sigal, E., Särkioja, T., Witztum, J.L. and Steinberg, D. (1991) J. Clin. Invest. 87, 1146–1152
87. Belkner, J., Wiesner, R., Rathman, J., Barnett, J., Sigal, E. and Kühn, H. (1993) Eur. J. Biochem. 213, 251–261
88. Belkner, J., Wiesner, R., Kühn, H. and Lankin, V.Z. (1991) FEBS Lett. 279, 110–114
89. Kühn, H., Belkner, J., Wiesner, R., Schewe, T., Lankin, V.Z. and Tikhaze, A.K. (1992) Eicosanoids 5, 17–22

4

Free radicals in the vasculature: pathological and physiological significance

Victor Darley-Usmar*, Neil Hogg†, Balaraman Kalyanaraman† and Kevin Moore‡

*Wellcome Research Laboratories, Beckenham, Kent BR3 3BS, U.K., †Biophysics Research Institute, Medical College of Wisconsin, 8701 Watertown Plank Road, Milwaukee, Wisconsin 53226, U.S.A. and ‡Department of Clinical Pharmacology, Royal Postgraduate Medical School, Du Cane Road, London W12 0NN, U.K.

Introduction

The vasculature is composed of a number of different cell types and constitutes one of the most important organs in the body. It is not surprising, therefore, that dysfunction of the biochemical processes in vascular cells is associated with the pathology of a number of human diseases. Among these are atherosclerosis, endotoxaemia and some aspects of ischaemia–reperfusion. In this short overview we will consider the several different roles of free radicals in the vasculature and, an aspect that is often overlooked, the role of free radicals under 'normal' conditions and their probable biological function. Particular emphasis will be placed on the chemical characteristics of the interactions between oxidants in the vasculature and their possible relevance to human disease.

The transfer of electrons is central to many biological processes and the biology of the vasculature is, of course, no exception. Free radicals usually result from the transfer of single electrons to or from biological molecules (reduction or oxidation) and have long been recognized as essential intermediates in many biological electron-transfer systems; for example, the formation of the ubisemiquinone radical from ubiquinol is essential for mitochondrial electron transfer. A more recent finding is that free radicals may also play a

*To whom correspondence should be addressed.

role as biological messengers and are capable of activating specific signal-transduction pathways. In some cases, free radicals have been implicated in the pathology of disease.

The role of the free radical nitric oxide (NO) in controlling vascular tone and the significance of its reaction with superoxide is currently attracting much interest. We will explore these areas in some detail, with particular emphasis on their possible contribution to the pathology of atherosclerosis. In addition, the controlled oxygenation of lipids by the lipoxygenase and cyclo-oxygenase enzymes has long been recognized for its role in producing potent mediators of inflammation. It now appears that non-specific lipid peroxidation products may also have important biological functions and the implications of these findings will be considered. What we hope will become evident is that, while our understanding of the role of free radicals in the vasculature is still in its infancy, their potential contribution to both normal and pathological conditions is immense and they should therefore continue to be of great interest.

Formation of free radicals in the vasculature

Nitric oxide

NO is produced *in vivo* by a family of enzymes, the NO synthases, which are found in a wide variety of cell types [1–3]. This free radical acts as a signal in the vasculature and nervous system and as a mediator of the cytotoxic action of macrophages [4–6]. NO synthases catalyse the oxidation of the guanido-N of arginine to generate citrulline and NO in an NADPH- and oxygen-dependent process [1,2,6]. The enzymes are homologous to cytochrome *P*-450 reductase and contain a number of redox centres, including haem, tetra-hydrobiopterin, FMN and FAD [7–9]. Once formed, NO diffuses from the cell to exert its biological effect. The different types of NO synthase enzyme and their control reflect the various roles of this free radical in biology. Several excellent reviews are available describing the biological actions and biosynthesis of NO and these aspects will not be covered in any detail here [1–3,10].

Under normal conditions in the vasculature, NO plays a key role in modulating vascular tone and is identical to endothelium-derived relaxing factor (EDRF), a molecule released by endothelial cells upon stimulation by vasodilators such as acetylcholine [4,11,12]. In this instance, NO is produced by a constitutive form of NO synthase, whose activity is calcium and calmodulin dependent [13,14]. The enzyme may be partially membrane bound and, once formed, NO diffuses from its site of formation and activates the soluble guanylate cyclase in arterial wall smooth muscle cells, causing an increase in production of cyclic GMP which ultimately results in muscle relaxation [15,16]. In marked contrast, the NO synthase of inflammatory cells, such as macrophages, is non-constitutive, calcium independent and can be induced by cytokines such as tumour necrosis factor (TNF) and interferon γ (IFN-γ) [6,9,10,17,18]. Inducible NO synthase can also be expressed in vascular smooth muscle cells, which may have important implications for the pathophysiology of septic shock. This inducible form of the enzyme is capable of generating a high flux of NO which exerts cytotoxic effects on both the generating cell and the target [10]. Although the cellular distribution of inducible NO synthase in human tissues is currently unclear, and, furthermore, the conditions required for its activation are not completely understood, it is likely to play an important role in human pathophysiology [19,20].

While it is established that NO is formed biologically and is a ligand and activator of guanylate cyclase, considerable interest has been aroused by the proposal that an S-nitrosothiol (e.g. glutathione S-NO, cysteine S-NO or serum albumin S-NO) may be formed *in vivo* and perform some, as yet undetermined, function [21,22]. Indeed, a nitrosylated thiol on human albumin has been detected *in vivo* [23]. It has been suggested that a nitrosothiol may in fact be EDRF but this appears unlikely (see [3]). These NO derivatives may take part in transnitrosation reactions and so modify thiols on proteins and perhaps change their biochemical function. Of particular importance to cardiovascular disease is the finding that a wide range of S-nitrosothiols and NO itself are able to inhibit platelet aggregation and adhesion to endothelial cells by elevating cyclic GMP levels [24–27]. Whether the effects of nitrosothiols occur through a direct transnitrosation reaction, which is unlikely since most of these compounds cannot penetrate the platelet membrane, or whether they are metabolized to release NO by a membrane-bound enzyme remains uncertain [26,28]. A similar mechanism has been proposed involving protein S-nitrosothiol formation for control of the function of the NMDA (N-methyl-D-aspartate) receptor, so modulating calcium fluxes in glutamate-stimulated neurons [29]. If S-transnitrosation is a biologically relevant control mechanism, in either platelets or the central nervous system, then it could be anticipated that specific enzymic processes exist to control the formation and reactivity of the S-nitrosothiols. The idea that thiol oxidation states may be used as a means to control intracellular metabolism is precedented by the example of the redox equilibrium between reduced and oxidized glutathione and the glutathione–protein thiol mixed disulphide [30].

Homolytic scission of the S-nitrosothiol to release NO and a thiyl radical by a light- and pH-sensitive reaction which is also susceptible to transition metal catalysis may also occur, and, in this case, it is likely that the thiyl radical will lead to the formation of superoxide or undergo other pro-oxidant reactions [31]. Clearly, the biology and chemistry of S-nitrosothiols will be of interest over the next few years. In the next two sections we will discuss some of the pro- and antioxidant reactions of NO.

NO as an antioxidant

In principle, NO could act as an antioxidant by (i) directly scavenging or inactivating oxidants which are formed *in vivo*, (ii) its action as a biological messenger, inhibiting the expression of enzyme systems responsible for generating oxidants, or (iii) directly inhibiting enzymes which are capable of generating oxidants. Experimental evidence consistent with these possibilities has been reported in the literature and is outlined below.

One effective method for inhibiting radical-dependent chain reactions is termination of the propagating radical with another radical species yielding a non-radical product: a reaction which NO could, in principle, undergo. A well-known and biologically relevant example of such a propagation reaction is lipid peroxidation, in which the lipid-centred peroxyl radical propagates a chain reaction. The reaction of organic peroxyl radicals with NO has been described under physiological conditions and estimated to occur at a rate of $1–3 \times 10^9 \, M^{-1}s^{-1}$ [32]. The product formed is presumably chemically related to peroxynitrite, as shown in the reaction below where ROO˙ represents an organic peroxyl radical.

$$ROO˙ + ˙NO \rightarrow ROONO$$

The rate of this reaction is far greater than that for the propagation of lipid peroxidation (see below), in which a hydrogen atom is extracted from an unsaturated fatty acid at a rate of approximately $10^2 \, M^{-1}s^{-1}$ [33].

$$ROO˙ + RH \rightarrow R˙ + ROOH$$

Since the inhibition of lipid peroxidation in human low-density lipoprotein (LDL) by NO was demonstrated it is clear that the organic peroxynitrite (ROONO) is not decomposing to form free radicals to any significant extent [34]. The products formed are still unknown but could be products of a rearrangement reaction such as an organic nitrate. The steady-state concentration of NO in the vasculature may be as high as $0.1 \, \mu M$ [35]. Since we know the rate of scavenging of peroxyl radicals by α-tocopherol ($5 \times 10^5 \, M^{-1}s^{-1}$), and also its approximate concentration in plasma ($25 \, \mu M$), we can compare its efficiency as an antioxidant with NO [36]. Under these conditions, the rate of scavenging of ROO˙ by NO is $(0.1 \times 10^{-6}) \times 10^9 = 100$ and for α-tocopherol is $(25 \times 10^{-6}) \times (5 \times 10^5) = 12.5$, suggesting that NO may play a significant role in suppressing lipid peroxidation in the vasculature. Such an effect could be further enhanced by the higher solubility of NO in the lipid phase of the LDL particle. The biological significance of this antioxidant reaction of NO is not known although it is consistent with an anti-atherogenic role for NO as will be discussed later.

NO is a ligand for both Fe (II) and Fe (III) and it is suggested that

NO may bind to and inhibit the iron-dependent redox cycles central to a number of mechanisms that create powerful oxidants [37,38]. One such mechanism is the reaction of haem proteins with hydrogen peroxide [38,39]. This results in the formation of the ferryl oxidation state of the haem iron which is a powerful oxidizing agent [40–42]. NO is able to act as a ligand to haem proteins and so inhibit the formation of ferryl myoglobin and thus inhibit haem-dependent lipid peroxidation. Likewise, NO may also inhibit the iron-dependent Fenton reaction and the consequent formation of hydroxyl radicals [38]. In addition to interactions with iron, NO was shown to inhibit the u.v.-dependent generation of hydroxyl radicals from hydrogen peroxide [38]. This reaction can proceed under anaerobic conditions and is not dependent on the presence of transition metals. The most likely explanation for the observed effects of NO in inhibiting this reaction are that it is able to scavenge hydroxyl radicals, although a direct reaction with hydrogen peroxide cannot be ruled out [43]. However, it is important to recognize that the extreme reactivity of the hydroxyl radical with biological targets precludes effective scavenging by NO *in vivo*. It is clear from the reactions described above, that hydrogen peroxide is an essential precursor in forming either the ferryl form of myoglobin or the hydroxyl radical via the Fenton reaction. The dismutation of superoxide is a major source of hydrogen peroxide in biological systems. The reaction of superoxide with NO may, therefore, inhibit both dismutation and the formation of oxidants via a hydrogen peroxide-dependent mechanism. The rate constant for the reaction between NO and superoxide is 6.7×10^9 M^{-1}s^{-1} at 37°C, compared with the rate constant for the spontaneous dismutation of superoxide of approx. 10^5 M^{-1}s^{-1} [44]. The data suggest that NO would also effectively scavenge superoxide if formed simultaneously within a given biological environment and thus inhibit the formation of hydrogen peroxide from superoxide. This hypothesis seems to be borne out by experiments with both NO donors and cells [45–47]; for example, it has been shown that superoxide formation from activated human leucocytes can be inhibited by NO [47]. This result prompted some authors to propose that NO has 'a cytoprotective role' as scavenger of the cytotoxic oxygen-derived free radical, superoxide [48]. However, this view asserts that the product of the reaction between NO and superoxide is itself inert. This is probably not the case as will be discussed later.

A number of enzymes, such as the lipoxygenases and cyclo-oxygenases, also contain iron which takes part in a redox cycle to catalyse reactions such as the oxygenation of lipids [49]. The activities of these enzymes are inhibited by NO when in a purified form [37]. Nevertheless, in intact cells, cyclo-oxygenase activity is apparently enhanced by NO [50]. This type of observation has generally been ascribed to the ability of a compound to protect the enzyme from inactivation mediated by lipid-derived radicals and is possibly the case here, since, as discussed previously, NO is a potent inhibitor of lipid peroxidation [32,34]. It is difficult to predict the outcome of the reactions of NO with the many ligands that could be present in the cell; however, it is important to bear in mind that the concentration of NO is generally low in the cell and that most of the potential binding sites have other ligands present at high concentration. It follows, therefore, that interactions which are chemically feasible may not always occur biologically.

Nitric oxide as a pro-oxidant

Two ideas have been discussed in this context. First, there is now good evidence to show that the non-specific cytotoxicity of activated murine macrophages is mediated directly by NO [10]. This may be of particular significance in the killing of parasites and, perhaps, tumour cells [10,51]. Since this reaction can also occur under anaerobic conditions, it is unlikely to involve oxygen, either directly or indirectly, or any of the products of NO with oxygen, e.g. nitrogen dioxide [10]. The mechanism of cell toxicity appears to involve the direct interaction of NO with electron-transfer proteins in the cell which contain iron–sulphur clusters, for example, aconitase and several electron-transfer proteins essential for the normal functioning of mitochondria [52]. These particular redox sites react with NO to form an inactive iron–nitrosyl complex and this is associated with the mobilization of iron from the cell [10]. However, these effects only occur when cells are exposed to high levels of the free radical and are only cytotoxic under conditions of low glucose [10]. The importance of direct NO-mediated cytotoxicity in the vasculature remains unclear.

The second idea is that NO acts as a precursor to the formation of oxidants such as peroxynitrite, nitrogen dioxide and the hydroxyl radical [53,54]. These mechanisms will be discussed in the section entitled Nitric oxide, oxygen and superoxide.

Superoxide

The one-electron reduction of oxygen yields the free radical superoxide, which may be formed in biological systems by a number of redox proteins within cells [55–59]. It has long been thought that the formation of this species occurs in a concerted and purposeful fashion in relatively few of these electron-transfer systems, one of which is the NADPH oxidase of the activated neutrophil [60]. In contrast, its generation during electron transfer in the mitochondria is thought to be accidental and potentially deleterious [58,59].

Despite the fact that the possible role of superoxide as a cytotoxic agent or extracellular messenger remains unresolved, we feel that both aspects are of sufficient interest to warrant discussion in the next sections. Although superoxide is clearly generated in the vasculature, it is fair to say that, unlike NO, the origin of superoxide has not been determined.

Superoxide as a cytotoxic agent

The widespread occurrence in biology of the enzyme superoxide dismutase (SOD), which catalyses the dismutation of the superoxide anion, has led to the hypothesis that this radical is toxic or that it leads to the formation of toxic metabolites [55–57]. Superoxide is not able to diffuse across biological membranes since it is charged at physiological pH. The SOD enzyme exists in a number of different forms which presumably serve different functions. For example, the mitochondrion, a major source of superoxide radicals within the cell, possesses a manganese-containing SOD. In this context, it is interesting to note that extracellular forms of SOD have also been described. There are three types, A, B and C, with type C having the highest affinity for heparin-binding sites on the endothelium [61]. An admittedly teleological argument suggests that extracellular SOD-C may have evolved to prevent the formation of peroxynitrite in the artery wall. In support of this idea, extracellular SOD-C is distributed throughout the interstitium and prevents the superoxide-dependent loss of EDRF activity in isolated rabbit aortic rings [61].

Investigation of the chemical properties of superoxide has revealed that the radical is not particularly reactive with biological molecules, which leads to the proposal that it may act as an intermediate for more powerful oxidants [55–57]. A plausible candidate for this role is the hydroxyl radical, which may be generated from superoxide and hydrogen peroxide in a sequence of reactions dependent on the presence of a transition metal catalyst, such as iron, and often referred to as the Fenton reaction, or by a transition-metal-independent reaction involving NO [53–56].

Possible sources of superoxide in the vasculature are (i) the NADPH oxidase of neutrophils, which generates superoxide on the outside of the plasma membrane and contains a b-type cytochrome as well as a number of other redox centres which are assembled prior to activation and superoxide generation, and (ii) the enzyme xanthine oxidase [56,60]. The role of xanthine oxidase under normal conditions is not clear; however, in ischaemia there is a rapid accumulation of purine metabolites, including hypoxanthine and xanthine, which are substrates for the enzyme. The enzyme can apparently exist in two forms, xanthine oxidase or xanthine dehydrogenase, using oxygen or NAD, respectively, as an electron acceptor [56]. It was originally thought that the dehydrogenase form of the enzyme was converted to the oxidase form after ischaemia in cardiac tissue [56], but this now appears unlikely [62,63]. When oxygen is used as an electron acceptor, the partial reduction of oxygen under these conditions results in the direct formation of both superoxide and hydrogen peroxide. The potential role of xanthine oxidase in mediating reperfusion damage in the myocardium has been extensively reviewed [56,64] and it is now clear that the presence of the enzyme is not necessary for reperfusion damage to occur. Some species, such as the rabbit, show all the characteristics of an oxygen-dependent dysfunction on reperfusion of ischaemic tissue without detectable xanthine oxidase activity in the heart [63]. Even in the rat, in which reasonable amounts of the enzyme have been detected, it now appears unlikely that it makes a significant contribution to tissue damage [62]. Nevertheless the contribution of xanthine oxidase to superoxide generation in other vascular beds cannot be ruled out [65].

Superoxide as a messenger in the vasculature

When cells form complex organs it is important that they can 'sense' the oxygen tension to which they are exposed, so that this information may be translated to control of other physiological functions. For this to occur, the cell requires an oxygen-sensing system and it is possible that the enzymic formation of superoxide may play just such a role. The amounts of superoxide produced are likely to be small and intracellular, but will vary according to the oxygen tension experienced by the cell in its local environment. The secondary messenger pathways mediating such effects remain obscure but could involve oxidation of the glutathione redox couple generated after increased superoxide formation [30].

Since the discovery of the role of the free radical NO as an intercellular messenger in the vasculature, it has been suggested that superoxide may also play a part in the control of vascular tone. Superoxide is in effect an NO antagonist, thus a role as endothelium-derived contracting factor has been proposed [66]. In support of this idea, a form of extracellular SOD (see section entitled Superoxide as a cytotoxic agent) has been found distributed throughout the intima of the artery and the rates of reaction of superoxide with either SOD or NO suggest that control by this mechanism is feasible [44,61]. However, since the product of the reaction, peroxynitrite, is a powerful oxidant it seems unlikely that nature would have selected such a potentially hazardous control mechanism.

Interactions between oxidants

Many potentially oxidizing species, some of which have been described above, have been detected or postulated to be present in the vasculature under both normal and pathological conditions. In this section we will discuss the interactions of vascular oxidants that may lead to an increase in oxidative stress.

Transition metals and peroxides

One widely entertained mechanism for the generation of hydroxyl radicals *in vivo* is the reaction known as the Fenton reaction (or sometimes the metal-ion-catalysed Haber–Weiss reaction). (For a brief discussion see section entitled Nitric oxide as an antioxidant.) This reaction involves the one-electron reduction of hydrogen peroxide by suitably chelated ferrous ions. The chemistry, biological occurrence and physiological significance of this reaction has been extensively reviewed and will not be discussed further [55].

A reaction that is in many ways analogous to the Fenton reaction involves the breakdown of lipid hydroperoxides by transition metal ions (principally iron and copper). The reduced form of the transition metal ion will react with lipid hydroperoxide to generate a lipid alkoxyl radical and the oxidized metal ion [67–69]. The alkoxyl radical is then able to extract a hydrogen atom from a neighbouring unsaturated fatty acid, thus initiating lipid peroxidation [67–69]. However, lipid peroxidation can be initiated by addition of the oxidized form of the metal ion only, demonstrating that either the oxidized metal ion itself can initiate lipid peroxidation or that the metal is being reduced by some other component of the experimental system. In this case, a redox cycle of the transition metal ion has been proposed to explain the catalytic role of metals in the promotion of lipid peroxidation. This mechanism of initiation of lipid peroxidation has been reviewed [67,68].

Transition metal ion oxidation of lipids has been extensively studied in the copper-dependent oxidation of LDL [69]. Copper will modify LDL to a form recognized by the macrophage scavenger receptor, which may be relevant to atherosclerosis (see section entitled Atherosclerosis). This mechanism probably does not occur under normal conditions *in vivo* since transition metals are generally sequestered by proteins in a form that cannot sustain this type of reaction. However, tissue damage may release iron and copper in a form that is capable of catalysing these reactions [70,71].

Haem-bound iron has also been observed to be a potent catalytic initiator of lipid peroxidation, either as haemoglobin, haemin or myoglobin [37–42,72,73]. These reactions may involve ferrous, ferric and/or ferryl forms of the haem iron and it may be postulated that a one-electron redox cycle of haem-bound iron has the potential to decompose lipid hydroperoxide by a mechanism similar to the one proposed for copper.

Nitric oxide, oxygen and superoxide

The characteristics of the reaction of NO with oxygen in solution have been described in some detail and it is now clear that, at physiological concentrations, the reaction between these gases proceeds at a negligible rate [74]. However, under physiological conditions, the biological half-life of EDRF or NO is decreased to 2–4 s suggesting that some other component is reacting with NO. The superoxide anion is a likely candidate since SOD enhances the effect of EDRF on tissue relaxation *in vitro* [66,75,76]. Indeed, as mentioned previously, this has prompted speculation about the role of superoxide in controlling the efficacy of EDRF [66,77,78] and generated interest in the physiological consequences of the reaction between NO and superoxide. Superoxide and NO may be generated simultaneously in vascular tissue or by inflammatory cells. The product of the reaction, peroxynitrite, has in fact been detected after activation of rat alveolar macrophages with phorbol ester [79–81]. NO and superoxide combine to form peroxynitrite, as shown in eqn. 1 [82], at a rate that is essentially diffusion controlled [32].

$$NO + O_2^- \rightarrow ONOO^- \tag{1}$$

The chemistry of peroxynitrite is complex [83]; however, it is clear that peroxynitrite is both an oxidant in its own right and is also able to exhibit many of the properties of the hydroxyl radical at pH 7.4. Peroxynitrite is thus a potentially deleterious oxidant in biological systems (eqn. 2).

$$ONOOH \rightarrow OH^\cdot + NO_2 \tag{2}$$

The free radical nature of peroxynitrite decomposition was more recently confirmed using an array of detection methods for hydroxyl radicals [53]. Chemical reactivity characteristic of hydroxyl radicals was also observed when NO and superoxide were generated simultaneously [45,54].

This includes the ability to oxidize deoxyribose or dimethylsulphoxide to malondialdehyde or formaldehyde respectively, or hydroxylate sodium benzoate [45,53,54]. Although these reactions are characteristic of the hydroxyl radical, it does not necessarily follow that 'free' hydroxyl radicals are released into solution. An alternative hypothesis is that peroxynitrite may exist in either a *cis* or *trans* conformation. In the *trans* configuration a transition state in an activated form is postulated, which will react in the vicinity of a target molecule as though it were a free hydroxyl radical [83]. This rather complex argument rests largely upon thermodynamic considerations and one might be tempted to take a rather more pragmatic view regarding the free radical nature of peroxynitrite decomposition. Put crudely, if it quacks, has wings and answers to the name Donald, it is probably a duck rather than a chicken in drag. However, the hydroxyl radical is so reactive that, in its 'free' form, it is likely to dissipate itself in an indiscriminate reaction with the nearest available molecule. In biological terms, the chance of such a reaction having any serious consequences is remote. The diffusion of a relatively stable molecule, such as peroxynitrite, presents an altogether more serious hazard since it may react with more critical targets necessary for biological function. Among these are tyrosine and cysteine, which react with peroxynitrite by a different mechanism to that described above. In the former case, the reactive intermediate is a nitrating agent, probably the nitryl cation (NO^{2+}), the formation of which can be catalysed by transition metals.

Interestingly, it was recently discovered that the copper centre of SOD can also promote phenol nitration by peroxynitrite, and, in the absence of exogenous phenols, a tyrosine residue of the enzyme was shown to be nitrated [84]. SOD-promoted phenol nitration has been used to detect the generation of peroxynitrite in cytokine-stimulated macrophages [80]. Thus, peroxynitrite represents part of the bactericidal armoury of the macrophage and has also been implicated in the NO-dependent killing of nerve cells [29,85].

The relevance of peroxynitrite *in vivo* has yet to be firmly established. However, the reaction of NO with superoxide, like the Fenton reaction, represents a mechanism in which 'leakage' from normal metabolic processes, and subsequent generation of superoxide, leads to the formation of a powerful and potentially deleterious oxidant.

Pathological implications

Atherosclerosis

Atherosclerosis is a disease of the artery wall associated with the formation of fat-filled or 'foam' cells largely derived from macrophages [86–91]. It is thought that oxidative modification of LDL within the artery wall ultimately leads to the formation of an atherosclerotic lesion and much evidence has accumulated to support this idea [90,92]. The nature and source of the oxidative stress is, however, largely unknown. One suggestion is that transition metals acting in concert with enzymes such as lipoxygenase may act to promote LDL oxidation [92,93]. While a role in advanced atherosclerotic lesions does seem likely (see later), it is nevertheless difficult to envisage the presence of free iron or copper in the pre-atherosclerotic artery and it is likely that the initiation of an atherosclerotic lesion is a transition metal ion-independent process.

Could the reaction between NO and superoxide to form peroxynitrite within the vasculature be an initial pro-atherosclerotic event as we have recently proposed [45]? This reaction depends only on the activity of cells constitutive to the normal artery wall and is a transition metal-independent process [45,53,54].

Indirect evidence suggests that the reaction between superoxide and NO occurs in the vasculature *in vivo*. For example, it has been shown that treatment of the spontaneously hypertensive rat with a genetically engineered variant of the SOD enzyme, capable of binding to the endothelial cell, lowered the blood pressure of these animals [94]. Interestingly, it is clear that the production of NO in the atherosclerotic lesions of cholesterol-fed rabbits is significantly elevated when compared with formation from normal regions of artery [95,96]. Furthermore, this is associated with an increased formation of superoxide, possibly derived from xanthine oxidase, and a lowered response of these vessels to EDRF-dependent relaxation [97]. A further study showed that treatment of cholesterol-fed animals with a modified form of SOD partially restored the endothelium-dependent response of the vasculature [97,98]. This result is consistent with a cytotoxic effect of superoxide in atherosclerotic lesions. Finally, a series of experiments *in vitro* have shown that the activation of soluble guanylate cyclase by NO is inhibited by oxidized LDL [99,100]. This form of LDL is cytotoxic and is thought to play a major role in initiating the atherosclerotic lesion [92]. It appears likely, therefore, that superoxide and NO are formed simultaneously within the artery wall, particularly in atherosclerotic lesions.

The effects of simultaneous generation of NO and superoxide on the potential atherogenicity of LDL have been investigated. Both these free radicals are unable to oxidize LDL alone; however, when generated simultaneously at approximately equal rates many of the phenomena associated with LDL oxidation were observed [45]. These include lipid peroxidation, α-tocopherol depletion, decrease of reactive amino groups and an increase in electrophoretic mobility [101–103]. The interaction of peroxynitrite with LDL also shows many of these characteristics and generates a form of the lipoprotein that is recognized and taken up by the macrophage scavenger receptor [103]. The uptake of LDL by the macrophage scavenger receptor represents a probable route of foam cell formation during atherogenesis [89]. Treatment of LDL with low concentrations of peroxynitrite increases its susceptibility to oxidation by transition metals such as copper [101].

In contrast, other investigators have studied the effect of NO on the cell-dependent modification of LDL in culture [104,105]. This experimental system employs monocultures of cells, typically macrophages, although other cell types have been used, in medium enriched with transition metals [91]. The system is thought to mimic some of the processes which may occur in the artery wall and which contribute to the development of an atherosclerotic lesion. Two research groups have shown that synthesis of NO is not required for the oxidative modification of LDL and, when induced, it inhibits the transition metal- and cell-dependent modification of the LDL particle [104,105]. This could occur by direct inhibition of the oxidant-generating mechanisms in this cell, for example a lipoxygenase enzyme, inhibition of the transition metal-dependent oxidation, or scavenging of peroxyl radicals (see also section entitled Nitric Oxide as an antioxidant). For the reasons discussed earlier, the relevance of these models to the early events in atherosclerosis is open to question. In these initial stages the key factor is likely to be the balance between superoxide- and NO-dependent generation in the artery wall. If more NO than superoxide is generated then, even if peroxynitrite is formed, this could be counteracted by the antioxidant activity of NO. This is consistent with the reported anti-atherogenic effects of L-arginine [106,107]. Alternatively, if more superoxide than NO is formed, the antioxidant function of NO will be lost and replaced by the pro-oxidant and potentially atherogenic reactions of peroxynitrite.

In more advanced lesions, iron or copper may play a role, as a consequence of metal release due to the oxidative damage of proteins such as transferrin or caeruloplasmin. This hypothesis is consistent with the presence of free iron and copper in advanced human atherosclerotic lesions [108]. Free iron or copper could then catalyse two oxidative processes: (i) the production of hydroxyl radicals from hydrogen peroxide via the Fenton reaction, and (ii) the initiation of lipid peroxidation within the LDL particle by the breakdown of endogenous lipid hydroperoxides (see section entitled Transition metals and peroxides). The second pathway requires a mechanism of 'seeding' LDL with lipid hydroperoxide, and in this context 15-lipoxygenase has been proposed [93].

Lipid oxidation products and vascular dysfunction

Lipid peroxidation may adversely affect cellular or tissue homoeostasis, either by alteration of integral lipids or by generation of lipid oxidation products which can alter cell function or viability directly. With the exception of LDL oxidation, it has been much more difficult to prove that any commonly studied markers of lipid peroxidation, namely the formation of malondialdehyde or the hydroxynonenals, have any relevance to disease pathology. On the other hand, epidemiological studies have indicated the possible beneficial effects of anti-oxidants in human disease [109,110]. One example of a class of non-specific lipid peroxidation products, the isoprostanes, will be used to illustrate the potential of lipid peroxidation to generate biological mediators capable of inducing vascular dysfunction.

Isoprostanes

The isoprostanes are formed as a direct consequence of the peroxidation of arachidonic acid via the generation of peroxyl radical isomers, which undergo endocyclization to prostaglandin (PG) G_2-like compounds and are subsequently reduced to PGF_2-like compounds [111].

The formation of these compounds *in vivo* was confirmed in two animal models of xenobiotic toxicity which clearly involve lipid peroxidation, namely diquat administration to selenium-deficient rats and carbon tetrachloride toxicity [111,112]. Administration of these compounds to the animals increased plasma levels of isoprostanes more than 200-fold, and this could not be inhibited by indomethacin. Moreover, recent studies by Morrow and colleagues (J.D. Morrow, personal communication) have shown that elevation in the formation of the F_2-isoprostanes can be enhanced by agents which deplete hepatic glutathione stores, such as phorone or buthionine sulphoximine, and agents which induce cytochrome P-450 (phenobarbitone or isonicotinic acid hydrazide) also enhance the elevation of plasma F_2-isoprostanes. There was also a commensurate increase in both hepatic (77-fold) and renal (15-fold) tissue levels of these compounds. Thus, there is good evidence to indicate that these compounds are formed *in vitro* and *in vivo* by a mechanism not involving cyclo-oxygenase.

A novel aspect of the mechanism of formation of these compounds is the fact that they may be formed as adducts to phospholipids in membranes. This is in contrast to enzymically generated prostanoids which are formed after cleavage of arachidonic acid from phospholipid [113].

One of the major isoprostanes formed in these animal studies was 8-epi-$PGF_{2\alpha}$. This is available in pure form and has been investigated for biological activity. When infused intrarenally at $0.5–2\,\mu g\,kg^{-1}min^{-1}$ it causes a dose-dependent reduction in glomerular filtration rate, with renal function ceasing at the highest dose. Furthermore, urinary excretion of these compounds increased by over 300% in a renal ischaemia–reperfusion model.

The isoprostanes are also active in other vascular beds; for example, studies in the rat and rabbit have indicated that 8-epi-$PGF_{2\alpha}$ is a potent pulmonary vasoconstrictor [114,115]. In the lung it is also a bronchoconstrictor, suggesting a potentially deleterious role in adult respiratory distress syndrome. These biological effects may be blocked by thromboxane receptor antagonists and are consistent with the action of 8-epi-$PGF_{2\alpha}$ as a partial agonist to the thromboxane receptor [114–117]. At present there are no published data on the effect of 8-epi-$PGF_{2\alpha}$ on the coronary vasculature, but it is likely to be a coronary vasoconstrictor and may, therefore, have an important role in reperfusion–vasoconstriction after procedures such as angioplasty.

To assess whether isoprostanes may be relevant in some human forms of acute renal failure in which lipid peroxidation may be important, studies have been carried out measuring plasma and urinary levels of F_2-isoprostanes in hepatorenal syndrome. This condition resembles a slow sepsis in which there is functional renal failure, with histologically normal kidneys, occurring as a consequence of renal vasoconstriction, and a decrease in the glomerular capillary ultrafiltration coefficient. A 10-fold increase in plasma levels of F_2-isoprostanes in hepatorenal syndrome, with normal levels in both liver disease controls and chronic renal failure, has been observed, suggesting that free radical injury occurs in this condition.

Sepsis

During sepsis there is increased synthesis of a variety of cytokines, activation of inflammatory cells, endothelial dysfunction, vasodilatation, increased microvascular permeability, and a variety of effects on lung, renal and hepatic function. Some of these processes may be directly linked to increased production of free radicals. Activation of inflammatory cells and platelets results in a respiratory burst and generation of the superoxide radical. Induction of NO synthase in vascular smooth muscle may result in vasodilatation and hypotension, and preliminary clinical studies using an inhibitor of NO synthase in patients with septic shock have been reported [118]. Interactions between oxidants may also play a role in inducing oxidative stress in septic shock. In support of an increase in oxidative stress during sepsis, animal studies have shown that a carbon-centred radical is formed in both liver and cardiac tissue 25 min after endotoxin administration [119]. Studies with the lazaroids (novel therapeutic oxidants with a broad range of properties) have demonstrated both increased survival of animals with experimental sepsis [120], and attenuated acute lung injury [121]. Likewise, administration of N-acetylcysteine, which increases the levels of the intracellular antioxidant glutathione, also decreases lung injury in endotoxin-treated rats [122]. The role of free radicals in the pathophysiology of sepsis is complex and multifactorial. It is likely to represent one area where therapeutic intervention with agents blocking the synthesis of free radicals (e.g. NO synthase inhibition) or improving host defence against generated free radicals (e.g. lazaroids, N-acetylcysteine) will improve survival in this group of patients.

Summary

What we now know about the mechanisms of electron transfer in the vasculature which lead to the production of oxidants suggests that their control is the key factor determining whether they contribute to the pathophysiology of disease. For example, we have proposed that in situations where NO is generated in excess over superoxide, the antioxidant action of NO may prevail over the pro-oxidant action of peroxynitrite. However, if superoxide is in excess then much of the NO will be converted to peroxynitrite and the reaction will be pro-oxidant. It follows, therefore, that the rates of generation of NO and superoxide in the vasculature may be critical in determining whether the artery wall is subjected to a pro- or antioxidant environment.

Once oxidants such as peroxynitrite are formed, the effects are likely to be highly dependent on the local environment. Modification of lipids can lead to eicosanoid-like substances, such as the isoprostanes or oxidized LDL, which may have long-ranging effects within the vasculature. Alternatively, modification of proteins may lead to direct effects on cell function. It is only when control of these interacting processes are lost that the consequences are likely to be pathological.

References
1.   Stuehr, D. and Griffith, O.W. (1992) Adv. Enzymol. **65**, 287–346
2.   Knowles, R.G. and Moncada, S. (1994) Biochem. J. **298**, 249–258
3.   Moncada, S., Palmer, R.M.J. and Higgs, E.A. (1991) Pharmacol. Rev. **43**, 109–142
4.   Palmer, R.M.J., Ferrige, A.G. and Moncada, S. (1987) Nature (London) **327**, 524–526
5.   Garthwaite, J., Charles, S.L. and Chess-Williams, R. (1988) Nature (London) **336**, 385–388
6.   Marletta, M.A., Yoon, P.S., Iyengar, R., Leaf, C.D. and Wishnok, J.S. (1988) Biochemistry **27**, 8706–8711
7.   Bredt, D.S., Hwang, P.M., Glatt, C.E., Lowenstein, C., Reed, R.R. and Snyder, S.H. (1991) Nature (London) **351**, 714–718
8.   White, K.A. and Marletta, M.A. (1992) Biochemistry **31**, 6627–6631
9.   Stuehr, D.J. and Ikeda-Saito, M. (1992) J. Biol. Chem. **267**, 20547–20550
10. Hibbs, J.B., Taintor, R.R. Vavrin, Z., Granger, D.L., Drapier, J.C., Amber, I.J. and Lancaster, J.R. (1990) in Nitric Oxide from L-arginine: A Bioregulatory System (Moncada, S. and Higgs, E.A., eds.), pp. 189–223, Elsevier, Amsterdam
11. Furchgott, F.R. (1984) Annu. Rev. Pharmacol. Toxicol. **24**, 175–197
12. Vallance, P., Collier, J. and Moncada, S. (1989) Lancet **ii**, 997–1000
13. Busse, R. and Mulsch, A. (1990) FEBS Lett. **265**, 133–136
14. Lopez-Jaramillo, P., Gonzalez, M.C., Palmer, R.M.J. and Moncada, S. (1990) Br. J. Pharmacol. **101**, 489–493

15. Förstermann, U., Schmidt, H.W., Pollock, J.S., Sheng, H., Mitchell, J.A., Warner, T.D., Nakone, M. and Murad, F. (1991) Biochem. Pharmacol. **42**, 1849–1857
16. Ignarro, L.J., Bush, P.A. and Buga, G.M. (1990) Biochem. Biophys. Res. Commun. **170**, 843–850
17. Hibbs, J.B., Taintor, R.R., Vavrin, Z. and Rachlin, E.M. (1988) Biochem. Biophys. Res. Commun. **157**, 87–94
18. Stuehr, D., Gross, S., Sakuma, I., Levi, R. and Nathan, C. J. (1992) Exp. Med. **169**, 1011–1020
19. Moncada, S. (1992) Acta. Physiol. Scand. **145**, 201–227
20. Denis, M. (1991) J. Leukocyte Biol. **48**, 380–387
21. Stamler, J.S., Simon, D.I., Osborne, J.A., Mullins, M.E., Jaraki, O., Michel, T., Singel, D.J. and Loscalzo, J. (1992) Proc. Natl. Acad. Sci. U.S.A. **89**, 444–448
22. Ignarro, L.J., Lipton, H., Edwards, J.C., Baricos, W.H., Hyman, A.L., Kadovitz, P.J. and Greutter, C.A. (1981) J. Pharmacol. Exp. Ther. **218**, 739–749
23. Keaney, J.F., Simon, D.I., Stamler, J.S., Jaraki, D., Scharfsein, J.,Vita, J.A. and Loscalzo, J. (1993) J. Clin. Invest. **91**, 1582–1589
24. Myers, P.R., Minor, R.L., Guerra, R., Bates, J.N. and Harrison, D.G. (1990) Nature (London) **345**, 161–163
25. Radomski, M.W., Palmer, R.M.J. and Moncada, S. (1987) Br. J. Pharmacol. **92**, 181–187
26. Radomski, M.W., Rees, D.D., Dutra, A. and Moncada, S. (1992) Br. J. Pharmacol. **107**, 745–749
27. Lieberman, E.H., O'Neill, S. and Mendelsohn, M. (1991) Circ. Res. **68**, 1722–1728
28. Kowaluk, E.A. and Fung, H.L. (1990) J. Pharmacol. Exp. Ther. **255**, 1256–1264
29. Lipton, S.A., Choi, Y.B., Pan, Z.H., Lei, S.Z., Chen, H.S., Sucher, N.J., Loscalzo, J., Singel, D.J. and Stamler, J.S. (1993) Nature (London) **364**, 626–632
30. Brigelius, R. (1985) in Oxidative Stress (Sies, H., ed.), pp. 243–272, Academic Press, London
31. Misra, H.P. (1974) J. Biol. Chem. **249**, 2151–2155
32. Padmaja, S. and Huie, R.E. (1993) Biochem. Biophys. Res. Commun. **195**, 539–544
33. Castle, L. and Perkins, M.J. (1986) J. Am. Chem. Soc. **108**, 6381–6382
34. Hogg, N., Kalyanaraman, B., Joseph, J. Struck, A. and Parthasarthy, S. (1993) FEBS Lett. **334**, 170–174
35. Malinski, T., Taha, Z., Grunfeld, S., Patton, S., Kapturezak, M. and Tomboulian, P. (1993) Biochem. Biophys. Res. Commun. **193**, 1076–1082
36. Niki, E., Saito, T., Kawakami, A. and Kamiya, Y. (1984) J. Biol. Chem. **259**, 4177–4182
37. Kanner, J., Harel, S. and Granit, R. (1992) Lipids **27**, 46–49
38. Kanner, J., Harel, S. and Granit, R. (1991) Arch. Biochem. Biophys. **289**, 130–136
39. Dee, G., Rice-Evans, C., Obeyesekara, S., Meraji, S., Jacobs, M. and Bruckdorfer, K.R. (1991) FEBS Lett. **294**, 38–42
40. Yusa, K. and Shikama, K. (1987) Biochemistry **26**, 6684–6688
41. Galaris, D., Sevianian, A., Cadenas, E. and Hochstein, P. (1990) Arch. Biochem. Biophys. **281**, 163–169
42. Kanner, J. and Harel, S. (1985) Arch. Biochem. Biophys. **237**, 314–321
43. Noronha-Dutra, A.A., Epperlein, M.M. and Woolf, N. (1993) FEBS Lett. **321**, 55–62
44. Huie, R.E. and Padmaja, S. (1993) Free Radical Res. Commun. **18**, 195–199
45. Darley-Usmar, V.M., Hogg, N., O'Leary, V.J., Wilson, M.T. and Moncada, S. (1992) Free Radical Res. Commun. **17**, 9–20
46. McCall, T.B., Boughton-Smith, N., Palmer, R.M.J., Whittle, B. and Moncada, S. (1989) Biochem. J. **261**, 293–296
47. Clancy, R.M., Leszczynska-Piziak, J. and Abramson, S.B. (1992) J. Clin. Invest. **90**, 1116–1121
48. Rabanyi, G.M., Ho, E.H., Cantor, E.H., Lumma, W.C. and Botehho, L.H.P. (1991) Biochem. Biophys. Res. Commun. **181**, 1392–1397
49. Yamamoto, S. (1992) Biochim. Biophys. Acta. **1128**, 117–131
50. Salvemini, D., Misko, T.P., Masterrer, J.L., Seibert, K., Currie, M.G. and Needleman, P. (1993) Proc. Natl. Acad. Sci. U.S.A. **90**, 7240–7244
51. Liew, F.Y., Millott, S., Parkinson, C., Palmer, R.M.J. and Moncada, S. (1990) J. Immunol.

144, 4707–4794
52. Lancaster, J.R. and Hibbs, J.B. (1990) Proc. Natl. Acad. Sci. U.S.A. **87**, 1223–1227
53. Beckman, J.S., Beckman, T.W., Chen, J., Marshall, P.A. and Freeman, B.A. (1990) Proc. Natl. Acad. Sci. U.S.A., **87**, 1620–1624
54. Hogg, N., Darley-Usmar, V.M., Wilson, M.T. and Moncada, S. (1992) Biochem. J., **281**, 419–424
55. Halliwell, B., and Gutteridge, J.M.C. (1986) Arch. Biochem. Biophys. **246**, 501–514
56. McCord, J.M. (1986) Adv. Free Radical Biol. Med. **2**, 325–345
57. Fridovich, I. (1986) Arch. Biochem. Biophys. **247**, 1–11
58. Nohl, H. and Jordan, W. (1986) Biochem. Biophys. Res. Commun. **138**, 533–539
59. Cadenas, E. and Boveris, A. (1980) Biochem. J. **188**, 31–37
60. Bellavite, P. (1988) Free Radical Biol. Med. **4**, 225–261
61. Abrahamsson, T., Brandt, U., Marklund, S. and Sjogvist, P.O. (1992) Circ. Res. **70**, 264–271
62. Kehrer, J.P., Piper, H.M. and Sies, H. (1987) Free Radical Res. Commun. **3**, 69–78
63. Downey, J.M., Miura, T., Eddy, L.J., Chambers, D.E., Nellert, T., Hearse, D.J. and Yellon, D.M. (1987) J. Mol. Cell. Cardiol. **19**, 1053–1060
64. Downey, J.M., Hearse, D.J. and Yellon, D.M. (1988) J. Mol. Cell. Cardiol. **20** (Suppl. II), 55–63
65. Panus, P.C., Wright, S.A., Chumby, P.H., Radi, R. and Freeman, B.A. (1992) Arch. Biochem. Biophys. **294**, 695–702
66. Katusic, Z.S. and Vanhoutte, P.M. (1989) Am. J. Physiol. **257**, H33–H37
67. Dix, T.A. and Aikens, J. (1993) Chem. Res. Toxicol. **6**, 2–18
68. Girotti, A. (1985) Free Radical Biol. Med., **1**, 87–95
69. Esterbauer, H., Gebicki, J., Puhl, H. and Jurgens, G. (1993) Free Radical Biol. Med. **13**, 341–390
70. Bolann, B.J. and Ulvik, R.J. (1987) Biochem. J. **243**, 55–59
71. Reif, D.W. and Simmons, R.D. (1993) Arch. Biochem. Biophys. **283**, 537–541
72. Szebeni, J., Winterbourn, C.C. and Carrell, R.W. (1984) Biochem. J. **220**, 658–692
73. Tappel, A.L. (1955) J. Biol. Chem. **217**, 721–733
74. Wink, D.A., Darbyshire, J.F., Nims, R.W., Saavedra, J.E. and Ford, P.C. (1993) Chem. Res. Toxicol. **6**, 23–27
75. Moncada, S., Palmer, R.M.J. and Gryglewski, R.J. (1986) Proc. Natl. Acad. Sci. U.S.A. **83**, 9164–9168
76. Gryglewski, R.J., Palmer, R.M.J. and Moncada, S. (1986) Nature (London) **320**, 454–456
77. Saran, M., Michel, C. and Bors, W. (1990) Free Radical. Res. Commun. **10**, 221–226
78. Halliwell, B. (1989) Free Radical Res. Commun. **5**, 315–318
79. McCall, T., Boughton-Smith, N.K., Palmer, R.M.J., Whittle, B.J. and Moncada, S. (1989) Biochem. J. **261**, 293–296
80. Ischiropoulos, H., Zhu, L. and Beckman, J.S. (1992) Arch. Biochem. Biophys. **298**, 446–451
81. Wang, J.F., Komarov, P., Sies, H. and DeGroot, H. (1991) Biochem. J. **279**, 311–314
82. Blough, N.V. and Zafiriou, O.C. (1985) Inorg. Chem. **24**, 3502–3504
83. Koppenol, W.H., Pryor, W.A., Moreno, J.J., Ischiropoulos, H. and Beckman, J.S. (1992) Chem. Res. Toxicol. **5**, 834–842
84. Smith, C.D., Carson, M., van der Woerd, M., Chen, J., Ischiropoulos, H. and Beckman, J.S. (1992) Arch. Biochem. Biophys. **299**, 350–355
85. Zhu, L., Gunn, C. and Beckman, J.S. (1992) Arch. Biochem. Biophys. **298**, 452–457
86. Schnaffner, T., Taylor, K., Bartucci, E.J., Fischer-Dzoga, K., Beeson, J.H., Glagov and Wissler, R.W. (1980) Am. J. Pathol. **100**, 57–73
87. Gerrity, R.G. (1981) Am. J. Pathol., **103**, 181–190
88. Brown, M.S. and Goldstein, J.L. (1983) Annu. Rev. Biochem. **52**, 223–261
89. Steinberg, D. (1988) Atheroscler. Rev. **18**, 1–23
90. Goldstein, J.L., Ho, Y.K., Basu, S.K. and Brown, M.S. (1979) Proc. Natl. Acad. Sci. U.S.A. **76**, 333–337
91. Esterbauer, H., Gebicki, J., Puhl, H. and Jurgens, G. (1993) Free Radical Biol. Med. **13**, 341–390
92. Parthasarathy, S., Wieland, E. and Steinberg, D. (1989) Proc. Natl. Acad. Sci. U.S.A. **86**, 1046–1050

93. Rankin, S.M., Parthasarathy, S. and Steinberg, D. (1991) J. Lipid Res. **32**, 449–456
94. Nakazono, K., Watanabe, N., Matsuno, K., Sasaki, J., Sato, T. and Inoue, M. (1991) Proc. Natl. Acad. Sci. U.S.A. **88**, 10045–10048
95. Minor, R.L., Myers, P.R., Guerra, R., Bates, J.N. and Harrison, D.G. (1990) J. Clin. Invest. **86**, 2109–2116
96. Ohara, Y., Peterson, T.E. and Harrison, D.G. (1993) J. Clin. Invest. **91**, 2541–2551
97. Mugge, A., Elwell, J.H., Peterson, T.E., Hofmeyer, T.G., Heistad, D.D. and Harrison, D.G. (1991) Circ. Res. **69**, 1293–1300
98. White, C.R., Brock, T.A., Chang, L.Y., Crapo, J., Briscoe, P., Ku, D., Bradley, W.A., Gianturco, S.H., Gore, J., Freeman, B.A., *et al.* (1994) Proc. Natl. Acad. Sci. U.S.A., **91**, 1044–1048
99. Schmidt, K., Graier, W.F., Kostner, G.M., Mayer, B., and Kukovetz, W.R. (1990) Biochem. Biophys. Res. Commun. **172**, 614–619
100. Chin, J.H., Azhar, S. and Hoffman, B.B. (1992) J. Clin. Invest. **89**, 10–18
101. Hogg, N., Darley-Usmar, V.M., Graham, A. and Moncada, S. (1993) Biochem. Soc. Trans. **21**, 358–362
102. Hogg, N., Darley-Usmar, V.M., Wilson, M.T. and Moncada, S. (1993) FEBS Lett. **326**, 199–203
103. Graham, A., Hogg, N., Kalyanaraman, B., O'Leary, V.J., Darley-Usmar, V. and Moncada, S. (1993) FEBS Lett. **330**, 181–185
104. Yates, M.T., Lamber, L.E., Whitten, J.P., McDonald, I., Mano, M., Ku, G. and Mao, S.J.T. (1992) FEBS Lett. **309**, 135–138
105. Jessup, W., Mohr, D., Geiseg, S.P., Dean, R.T. and Stocker, R. (1992) Biochem. Biophys. Acta. **1180**, 73–82
106. Drexler, H., Zeiher, A.M., Meinzer, K. and Just, H. (1991) Lancet **338**, 1546–1550
107. Cooke, J.P., Singer, A.H., Tsao, P., Zera, P., Rowan, R.A. and Billingham, M.E. (1992) J. Clin. Invest. **90**, 1168–1172
108. Smith, C., Mitchinson, M.J., Aruoma, O. and Halliwell, B. (1992) Biochem. J. **286**, 901–905
109. Rimm, E.B., Stampfer, M.J., Asherio, A., Giovannicc, E., Colditz, G.A. and Willett, W.C. (1993) N. Engl. J. Med. **328**, 1450–1456
110. Stampfer, M.J., Hennekens, C.H., Manson, J.E., Colditz, G.A., Rosner, B. and Willett, W.C. (1993) N. Engl. J. Med. **328**, 1444–1449
111. Morrow, J.D., Hill, K.E., Burk, R.F., Nammour, T.M., Badr, K.F. and Roberts II, L.J. (1990) Proc. Natl. Acad. Sci. U.S.A. **87**, 9383–9387
112. Morrow, J.D., Awad, J.A., Kato, T., Takahashi, K., Badr, K.F., Roberts II, L.J. and Burk, R.F. (1992) J. Clin. Invest. **90**, 2502–2507
113. Morrow, J.D., Awad, J.A., Boss, H.J., Blair, I.A. and Roberts II, L.J. (1992) Proc. Natl. Acad. Sci. U.S.A. **89**, 10721–10725
114. Kang, K.H., Morrow, J.D., Roberts II, L.J., Newman, J.H. and Banerjee, M. (1992) J. Appl. Physiol. **74**(1), 460–465
115. Banerjee, K., Kang, K.H., Morrow, J.D., Roberts, L.J. and Newman, J.H. (1992) Am. J. Physiol. **263**, H660–H663
116. Takahashi, K., Nammour, T.M., Fukunaga, M., Ebert, J., Morrow, J.D., Roberts, L.J., Hoover, R.L. and Badr, K.F. (1992) J. Clin. Invest. **90**, 136–141
117. Morrow, J.D., Minton, T.A. and Roberts II, L.J. (1992) Prostaglandins **44**, 155–163
118. Petros, A., Bennett, D. and Vallance, P. (1991) Lancet **338**, 1557–1558
119. Brackett, D.J., Lai, E.K., Lerner, M.R., Wilson, M.F. and McCay, P.B. (1989) Free Radical Res. Commun. **7**, 315–324
120. Powell, R.J., Machiedo, G.W., Rush, B.F. and Dikda, G.S. (1991) Am. Surg. **57**, 86–88
121. Tanigaki, T., Suzuki, Y., Heimer, D., Sussman, H.H., Ross, W.G. and Raffin, T.A. (1993) J. Appl. Physiol. **74**, 2155–2160
122. Feddersen, C.O., Barth, P., Puchner, A. and Von-Wichert, P. (1993) Med. Klin. **88**, 197–206

5

Cell-mediated oxidation of lipoproteins

Wendy Jessup* and David S. Leake†

*Cell Biology Group, Heart Research Institute, 145 Missenden Road, Camperdown, Sydney, NSW 2050 Australia and †School of Animal and Microbial Sciences, University of Reading, Whiteknights, PO Box 228, Reading, Berkshire, RG6 6AJ, U.K.

Introduction

Henriksen *et al.* [1] first described the ability of arterial endothelial cells to modify low-density lipoprotein (LDL) so that it was more rapidly endocytosed by macrophages. The dependence of this transformation on oxidation of the lipoprotein particle [2], and the ability of oxidized LDL (oLDL) to promote lipid loading in macrophages sufficient to develop a foam-cell phenotype [3], were the key observations which triggered an explosion of interest in lipoprotein oxidation. Since lipid oxidation products are also present in atheromatous tissues, lipoprotein oxidation is now widely believed to be involved in the pathogenesis of human atherosclerosis. This has been supported by epidemiological studies indicating an inverse correlation between antioxidant status and risk of cardiovascular disease, and animal studies in which antioxidant supplementation appears to inhibit the development of atherosclerotic lesions.

Most cell-mediated lipoprotein oxidation measured *in vitro* is dependent on the simultaneous presence of trace amounts of redox-active transition metals in the medium, and it should be assumed that all cell-mediated oxidation discussed in this chapter is metal-dependent, unless explicitly stated otherwise. The details of this dependence and its relevance to lipoprotein oxidation *in vivo* are discussed later.

The early studies concentrated on the ability of oLDL to promote lipid loading of macrophages, but over the intervening decade it has become clear that components of oLDL can also influence a number of other cellular functions which may be of relevance in atherogenesis. These include effects on the synthesis and secretion of mediators, expression of cell-surface molecules, chemotaxis, cell proliferation and cell viability. Despite the enormous interest in the role of lipoprotein oxidation in the pathology of atherosclerosis, however, it is still not clear how oxidized lipoproteins might be formed *in vivo*. The presence of a large antioxidant capacity in plasma [4] and the detection of only very low levels of peroxidation products in plasma lipoproteins [5] indicates that local oxidation of lipoproteins in the intima is probably the major route for their formation. The purpose of this chapter is to describe the mechanisms by which intimal cells may oxidize LDL *in vivo*. In addition, the metabolism of oLDL by cells and its effects on their function will be briefly reviewed.

Characteristics of cell-oxidized lipoproteins

The majority of studies of lipoprotein oxidation have been performed in cell-free systems in the presence of (relatively) high concentrations of transition metals, such as copper, since it is believed that this system largely mimics the cell-mediated LDL oxidation which has been observed *in vitro*. The chemical and functional changes which occur when LDL is oxidized in the presence of copper have been the subject of numerous reviews [6] and are covered elsewhere in this book (see Chapter 3 by Esterbauer, this volume). Although rather less attention has been given to the composition of cell-oxidized LDL, most studies indicate that these particles undergo a similar transformation *in vitro*. Thus, like LDL exposed to copper, cell-mediated oxidation of LDL sees (i) a loss of native cholesterol and cholesteryl esters and consumption of α-tocopherol [7], (ii) hydrolysis of phospholipids [2], (iii) formation of fatty acyl peroxidation products [8] and fragmentation of apolipoprotein B (apo B) [2], and (iv) generation of a number of oxysterols. The predominant oxysterol species generated by macrophages and copper oxidation are 7-ketocholesterol and 7β-hydroxycholesterol [9,9a], whereas in a study of endothelial cell-oxidized LDL only cholesterol α-epoxide was detected [10]. The difference between cell types may reflect the differences in the degree of oxidation achieved in each case; in metal-dependent cell-free oxidation, cholesteryl epoxides are generated early on in oxidation [11], whereas 7-ketocholesterol appears later and is more stable [12]. Though not yet exhaustively studied, many of the effects of cell-oxidized LDL on cellular function match those of copper-oxidized LDL (see later).

Lipoproteins sensitive to cell-mediated oxidation

In principle, any lipoprotein containing polyunsaturated fatty acids is susceptible to oxidation. Whether cells can be seen to initiate and/or promote this process will depend upon a number of factors, such as the sensitivity of the available detection methods, the antioxidant protection afforded to the lipoprotein and whether the cellular activity involves any degree of selectivity. For example, a requirement for direct physical contact between cell and LDL has been suggested, on the basis of limited early studies using a dialysis membrane to separate cells and lipoprotein [13]. More recently, binding to the LDL receptor for macrophage-mediated oxidation has been proposed [13a]. The biochemical basis of this apparent requirement for cell–LDL contact is not yet known, nor whether internalization (and subsequent retroendocytosis) of the lipoprotein particle is an essential component in the oxidative events which follow. Nevertheless, these preliminary studies indicate how cells could exert some selectivity in their oxidation of individual lipoprotein types.

The vast majority of the studies on oxidized lipoproteins have involved LDL [14–16], but other lipoproteins can also be oxidized by cells. Although high-density lipoprotein (HDL) and very-low-density lipoprotein (VLDL) are not transformed into avidly endocytosed species by endothelial cells [17,18], HDL lipids can be oxidized in the presence of endothelial cells [18]. β-Migrating VLDL (β-VLDL; a cholesterol-enriched remnant lipoprotein found in cholesterol-fed animals and in an uncommon form of human hyper-lipidaemia) is oxidized by rabbit [19] and bovine [20] endothelial cells. Lipoprotein(a) [Lp(a)] has been reported to be oxidized by macrophages to a form more rapidly endocytosed by fresh macrophages [21]. Carpenter *et al.* [22] have shown that coacervates of polyunsaturated fatty acids and albumin, used as a model for LDL, can be oxidized by monocyte-macrophages.

Cell types capable of lipoprotein oxidation

The first cell type shown to be capable of oxidizing LDL was a rabbit aortic endothelial cell line [1]. It has since been shown that human [23,24] and pig [24,25] aortic endothelial cells will also mediate LDL oxidation, as do human umbilical vein endothelial cells [17,23,24], human microvascular endothelial cells [23] and pig endocardial cells [25]. It was once thought that bovine aortic endothelial cells were not capable of oxidizing LDL; however, it has now been shown that they can do so but only slowly [25].

Guinea pig, pig, primate or human arterial smooth muscle cells can oxidize LDL [17,26,27], as can human peripheral blood lymphocytes [28,29], including CD4-positive cells, the main type of lymphocyte found in human atherosclerotic lesions [30].

Macrophages themselves can oxidize LDL; this has been shown for resident mouse peritoneal macrophages [31,32], human monocytes [33], human monocyte-derived macrophages [34,35], human blood mononuclear cells [36] and macrophage-derived foam cells isolated from rabbit atherosclerotic lesions [37]. Activated monocytes modify LDL to increase its uptake by endothelial cells *in vivo* and by endothelial cells in culture [38]. The LDL was incubated with the monocytes for only 30 min but the modification was inhibited by the antioxidant, α-tocopherol. Thus, all major cell types in atherosclerotic lesions are capable of oxidizing LDL. The macrophage is the most effective of these cells in oxidizing LDL [25,28], however, and may therefore play a key role in LDL oxidation in lesions.

Human neutrophils (which are rare in lesions) have been shown to oxidize LDL to make it cytotoxic to cells [33].

Mechanisms of cell-mediated LDL oxidation

General considerations

Cell-mediated lipoprotein oxidation has been most extensively studied *in vitro*, employing tissue culture systems in which the modifying cells are bathed with a medium containing the target lipoprotein. In most cases, oxidation is assessed by the assay of lipid oxidation products in an aliquot of supernatant. Early studies of cell-mediated LDL oxidation were often linked to measurements of functional changes in the lipoprotein, such as the development of toxic properties or its transformation into a scavenger receptor ligand. Although these, and particularly the latter, properties are still often used as biological endpoints for assay of cell-mediated oxidation, as the range of recognized biological effects of oLDL increases it is becoming more common to use more widely applicable measures of oxidation. This is still most often the TBARS (thiobarbituric acid-reactive substances) assay, although more sensitive and specific methods for direct determination of lipid peroxides have also been applied in a minority of cases. It is worth noting that only a small proportion ($\sim 20\%$ [39]) of LDL lipid peroxides generate TBA-reactive products during the TBARS assay. Also, the majority (>90%) of the TBARS detected in such supernatants are low molecular mass products which do not re-isolate with the LDL particle upon ultracentrifugation or ultrafiltration [40] and are presumably water-soluble lipid oxidation products. In some cases rather indirect assays can be quite informative, such as the particle net charge (measured by electrophoresis in agarose) and changes in epitopes on apo B.

The composition of the medium is an important factor in the extent of LDL oxidation which occurs in these systems [41,42]. The presence of trace (i.e. micromolar) amounts of redox-active metals appears, in all cases examined, to be an absolute requirement for cell-mediated LDL oxidation, based on the inhibitory effects of added metal chelators (EDTA, desferrioxamine, DTPA, hydroxypyridinones) [2,26,36,41,41a]. It has recently also been shown that LDL oxidation by macrophages occurs in a simple phosphate buffer containing added iron at acidic pH [43]. Of course this does not exclude the possibility that LDL oxidation *in vivo* is metal independent and some potential oxidative mechanisms which do not require metal catalysis have been described (see below).

It should be noted that the media which support cell-mediated oxidation are also capable of maintaining a finite rate of LDL oxidation in their own right [44], albeit at a slower rate than that measured when cells are present [7]. This cell-free oxidation has been reported to be dependent on the presence of low amounts of lipid peroxides in the starting LDL, since careful pretreatment of LDL with Ebselen plus glutathione (which reduces lipid hydroperoxide to lipid hydroxide) makes it resistant to such metal-catalysed oxidation (as judged by TBARS [45]). It has been suggested that lipid hydroperoxides act as reductants of Cu^{2+} and/or Fe^{3+}.

$$LOOH + M^+ \rightarrow LOO^{\cdot} + M + H^+ \tag{1}$$

This reaction is thermodynamically unfavourable [46], and cell-mediated oxidation might function by generating other, more efficient, cell-derived transition metal reductants (see below). The reduced metals are then (relatively) more capable of degradation of LOOH, with formation of secondary radicals that themselves can promote lipid peroxidation:

$$LOOH + Fe^{2+} \text{ (or } Cu^+) \rightarrow LO^{\cdot} + Fe^{3+} \text{ (or } Cu^{2+}) + OH^- \tag{2}$$
$$LO^{\cdot} + LH \rightarrow LOH + L^{\cdot} \tag{3}$$
$$L^{\cdot} + O_2 \rightarrow LOO^{\cdot} \tag{4}$$
$$LOO^{\cdot} + LH \rightarrow LOOH + L^{\cdot} \tag{5}$$

where LOOH = lipid hydroperoxide; $LO^{\cdot}$ = lipid alkoxyl radical; $L^{\cdot}$ = lipid radical; $LOO^{\cdot}$ = lipid peroxyl radical; and LH = lipid with bisallylic hydrogens. It is not yet clear if the presence of seeding levels of lipid peroxides is equally essential for cell-mediated oxidation of LDL. Supplementation of culture medium with Ebselen and glutathione largely inhibits macrophage-mediated oxidation [45], but this may be acting by retarding the rate of propagation of peroxidation in the particle rather than its initiation.

The most commonly used medium for cell-mediated oxidation is Ham's F-10, which contains both iron $(3 \mu M)$ and copper $(0.01 \mu M)$ in its formulation. MEM (no added metal), M199 $(0.25 \mu M$ Fe), RPMI-1640 (no added metal), and DMEM $(1.8 \mu M$ Fe) have also been used with varying success. For example, some groups found that RPMI does not support cell-mediated oxidation [2,47] while others found that it does [36,48]. Similarly, Leake and Rankin [41] found that DMEM $(1.8 \mu M$ Fe) does not permit detectable macrophage-mediated oxidation (measured indirectly by formation of high-uptake LDL), even in the presence of added $(3 \mu M)$ iron while Steinbrecher et al. [2] found that DMEM containing $5 \mu M$ Cu does allow extracellular-mediated oxidation. Even though RPMI and MEM have no transition metals in their formulation, it is possible that trace amounts are introduced as contaminants of reagents and water used during medium preparation [49]. We have recently noted (using a sensitive assay of LDL oxidation [12]) that cell-mediated oxidation which can be detected in Hanks' balanced salt solution, prepared using nanopure water, could be prevented by pretreatment of the solution with Chelex (L. Kritharides, W. Jessup and R.T. Dean, unpublished work), suggesting that adventitious metal contamination is the major factor in this system. Cathcart *et al.* [48] suggested that an additional source of transition metals may be the cells themselves.

The metal content is not the only component of the medium which affects cell-mediated oxidation rates. The presence of cysteine and/or cystine is also important (see below) but, in general, all the above media have comparable total amounts of these amino acids. Other variables include the content of antioxidant molecules, such as lipoic acid and phenol red [50].

The biochemical basis of the apparent pro-oxidant activity contributed by cells in LDL oxidation has been the subject of several studies, though no consensus yet exists on the true mechanism(s). From a theoretical standpoint a number of potential mechanisms can be proposed, including; (i) introduction of peroxides into LDL by direct action of enzymes or by transfer of peroxidized cellular lipids (e.g. by lipoxygenases); (ii) the direct action of cell-derived oxidants on the lipoprotein to initiate LDL peroxidation (e.g. superoxide radical, hydrogen peroxide, hypochlorite, reactive nitrogen species); (iii) provision and/or replenishment of extracellular reductant to maintain redox-active metal-catalysed oxidation at a maximum rate (e.g. by superoxide radical or reduced thiols); (iv) removal of endogenous lipoprotein antioxidants; and (v) generation of a local microenvironment favourable for metal-mediated oxidation (e.g. low pH).

The process of LDL oxidation can be considered as two separate stages: initiation and propagation. In such a scheme, cells might promote overall oxidation either by acting as initiators of the process (i.e. by formation of lipid radical species) or by maintaining or supplementing ongoing peroxidation either through the introduction of additional peroxides or by promoting metal-catalysed hydroperoxide decomposition.

Lipoxygenases

Lipoxygenases are enzymes which introduce peroxide groups into unsaturated fatty acids, and have been considered as potential agents for direct or indirect introduction of lipid peroxides into LDL by cells [13,24,51–53]. These enzymes are classified according to the position at which they introduce a hydroperoxide group into arachidonic acid (e.g. 5-,12- and 15-lipoxygenases), though they are also active with other fatty acid substrates to varying extents [54]. However, only mammalian (e.g. reticulocyte) 15-lipoxygenase is known to be able to oxidize esterified fatty acids, such as phospholipids in membranes [55] and cholesteryl esters in lipoproteins [56]. The direct action of such enzymes on LDL, or the release of lipoxygenase-derived lipid peroxyl radicals or hydroperoxides in the vicinity of the lipoprotein particle, might increase the peroxide content of LDL and the sensitivity of the particle to metal-catalysed oxidation. In agreement with this, O'Leary *et al.* [57] have shown that the direct addition of commercially available fatty acid hydroperoxides to LDL *in vitro* enhances its subsequent oxidation by copper.

The suggestion that lipoxygenase activity is an essential participant in cell-mediated LDL oxidation *in vitro* was initially based on the observed influence of lipoxygenase inhibitors added to the medium together with and/or prior to the lipoprotein. Most lipoxygenase inhibitors act either by metal chelation or peroxyl radical scavenging and as such are obviously not suitable agents for use in this metal-dependent peroxidation system. Some inhibitors remain which act by other mechanisms, including several 5-lipoxygenase inhibitors which prevent assembly of an active enzyme complex (e.g. MK886, Revlon 5901). Using these agents, we have shown that 5-lipoxygenase is not necessary for macrophage-mediated LDL oxidation [58]; this has since been confirmed by two independent groups [59,60].

ETYA (5,8,11,14-eicosatetraynoic acid) is an inhibitor of all lipoxygenases and has little or no intrinsic antioxidant activity. It does suppress LDL oxidation mediated by endothelial cells [13,24,60], monocytes [52] and macrophages [53,58,61], but quantitative studies indicate that the concentrations of ETYA which inhibit cell-mediated LDL oxidation do not match those which completely suppress cellular 15-lipoxygenase activity [24,58,60]. In addition, several groups have reported cytotoxic effects of ETYA in the same concentration range as inhibition of LDL oxidation [58,60–62] and while this has been suppressed by the addition of low amounts of serum in some cases [13,53,59], in others toxicity was still a significant problem [58,60,61].

There are presently no other lipoxygenase inhibitors available (other than for 5-lipoxygenase) which have been unequivocally shown to be free of antioxidant activity. RG 6866 (*N*-methyl-4-benzoxylphenylacetohydroxamic acid) inhibits monocyte-mediated [59] and endothelial cell-mediated [24] LDL oxidation, but, while the latter study reported no inhibitory effect of this compound on cell-free copper oxidation of LDL, in the former it was found to be a very efficient inhibitor of the same process. Piriprost and A64077 (*N*-(1-benzo(*b*)thien-2-ylethyl)-*N*-hydroxyurea) also suppress macrophage-mediated lipoprotein oxidation [53] but their enzyme specificities have not yet been rigorously examined and A64077 also inhibits cell-free copper oxidation of LDL [60].

The detection of active 15-lipoxygenase in atherosclerotic lesions [63] and the colocalization of immunoreactive 15-lipoxygenase and oLDL in the same regions of atherosclerotic plaques [64] are consistent with a function for lipoxygenases in local lipoprotein oxidation. One would predict that if cellular lipoxygenases have direct access to LDL during its oxidation, then in a metal-free medium stereospecific hydroperoxide products would accumulate in the lipoprotein. Alternatively, stereospecific fatty acid oxygenation products may be released from the cells and should be detectable either in the lipoprotein or the extracellular medium generally. Careful structural analysis of the oxygenated lipids from human atherosclerotic lesions [65] and LDL oxidized *in vitro* by endothelial cells [8] shows a non-specific product pattern indicative of predominantly non-enzymic oxidation, although in early lesions evidence of specific lipoxygenase products has recently been reported [65a]. Another consideration is that lipoxygenases are intracellular enzymes, and cells generally release hydroxy- rather than hydroperoxy-fatty acids on stimulation of cellular arachidonate metabolism as they have quite efficient peroxidases to reduce intracellular lipid hydroperoxides to more stable hydroxides [66]. Studies *in vivo* have failed to resolve the issue, since they have indicated the presence of only the hydroxides; furthermore, while levels of 15-hydroxy-5,8,11,13-eicosatetraenoic acid (15-HETE) [67] and 13-hydroxy-9,11-octadecadienoic acid (13-HODE) [68] were elevated in the intima of cholesterol-fed rabbits, a decreased formation of esterified 15-HETE and 13-HODE was measured in a similar experimental model. The issue of the role of lipoxygenases as agents of cell-mediated LDL oxidation therefore remains unresolved. Current studies using cells transfected with 15-lipoxygenase may provide the answer [68a,68b].

Superoxide radical

Superoxide radical ($O_2^{\cdot-}$) is secreted constitutively by most cell types to varying degrees and has been considered by many groups as a contributory agent in cell-mediated oxidation [69]. The radical itself is unable to induce peroxidation in unsaturated fatty acids in homogeneous solution [70] or in LDL [71], although superoxide treatment of LDL does induce a gradual consumption of endogenous α-tocopherol and sensitizes the particle to subsequent copper-mediated oxidation [71]. Superoxide generated enzymically by xanthine oxidase does not generate modified high-uptake LDL either [13], although protease contamination of many commercial preparations of this enzyme can lead to such extensive degradation of apo B (independently of the presence of xanthine substrate; S.P. Gieseg and W. Jessup, unpublished work) that any scavenger receptor ligands formed by the superoxide radical may possibly be destroyed. At low pH the protonated form, hydroperoxyl radical ($HO_2^{\cdot}$), is a much more powerful oxidant which can induce both tocopherol consumption and lipid peroxidation in LDL [71]. This may explain the observed acceleration of macrophage-mediated LDL oxidation at acidic pH [43]. However, neither superoxide nor hydroperoxyl radicals alone can convert LDL to a scavenger receptor ligand in a metal-free buffer [71].

In the presence of iron or copper, superoxide can generate hydroxyl radicals by the Fenton reaction [49]; these are very efficient oxidants of LDL [71]. However, hydroxyl radicals do not generate high-uptake LDL despite their peroxidative activity, and hydroxyl radical scavengers do not inhibit cell-mediated oxidation of LDL [23,27,36,71a,72], so perhaps a more probable function for the superoxide radical in cell-mediated oxidation would be as a reductant for Fe^{3+} and Cu^{2+}.

$$Fe^{3+} \text{ (or } Cu^{2+}) + O_2{}^{\cdot -} \rightarrow Fe^{2+} \text{ (or } Cu^+) + O_2 \qquad (6)$$

As such, superoxide could promote LDL oxidation according to reactions (2–5), driving the decomposition of lipid hydroperoxides within the LDL particle by efficiently maintaining the metals in their much more reactive reduced states.

The experimental basis for the hypothesis that superoxide radical is responsible for cell-mediated oxidation depends on two major sets of observations. The first rely on the inhibitory activity of superoxide dismutase (SOD). Many studies have shown that the addition of SOD can cause substantial inhibition of LDL oxidation by a number of cell types [27,36,47,48,50]. In fact, examination of these data indicate that the degree of inhibition of LDL oxidation is quite variable between studies, is usually incomplete, and in some cases SOD has no consistent inhibitory effect and can even promote LDL oxidation [71a]. This has led to the suggestion that the quantitative contribution of the superoxide radical to LDL oxidation varies between different cell types [69].

It has been known for some time that SOD also inhibits cell-free, copper-mediated LDL oxidation [13]. The reason for this is not clear, but could be explained by two recent studies [47,72a] which demonstrate that SOD can both chelate copper in a redox-inactive form and act as a peroxyl radical scavenger. Since the cell-mediated LDL oxidation in the systems studied using SOD is usually metal-dependent, the observed inhibitory activity of SOD may be due to its metal-binding ability rather than its catalytic dismutation of superoxide. Variabilities in the efficiency of inhibition of cell-mediated oxidation measured in the presence of SOD could depend on the relative amounts of SOD protein and redox-active metal present in each case. Our conclusion must therefore be that all studies involving the use of SOD as a test of superoxide involvement in cell-mediated LDL oxidation must be interpreted with caution.

More direct evidence for superoxide-dependent, cell-mediated oxidation has been obtained by Steinbrecher [50], who compared the ability of several different cell types (human skin fibroblasts, bovine aortic endothelial cells, rabbit arterial smooth muscle cells and rabbit endothelial cells) to oxidize LDL and found that the rates of LDL oxidation were directly correlated with their rates of cytochrome c-detectable superoxide output. Early studies with purified human monocytes indicated that these cells would only promote LDL oxidation in RPMI-medium when the cells were treated with stimuli such as opsonized zymosan, suggesting that respiratory burst-derived superoxide radical was involved [48]. However, LDL added to the cells as much as 6–8 h after zymosan (when the respiratory burst activity was complete) was apparently oxidized as efficiently as LDL added simultaneously with the stimulus, indicating that in this particular system zymosan operates by mechanisms other than stimulation of superoxide output, possibly related to metal contaminants present in zymosan. In contrast, Hiramatsu *et al.* [36] have shown that peripheral blood mononuclear cells (PBMC; ~30% monocytes/ 70% lymphocytes) oxidize LDL in RPMI in the absence of added stimuli, but that oxidation is increased when phorbol 12-myristate 13-acetate (PMA) is added to the cells. They suggest that this augmentation is due to the accompanying stimulation of superoxide output, and report that PBMC, from a chronic granulomatous disease patient (deficient in respiratory burst oxidase activity), treated with PMA oxidize LDL less efficiently than normal cells. However, this could not be confirmed in an independent study [35]. In addition, we have recently demonstrated that purified murine macrophages, stimulated with PMA or zymosan, oxidize LDL at the same rate as untreated cells. Similarly, PMA-stimulation of purified human monocyte-derived macrophages, while vastly enhancing superoxide output, had no accelerating effect on their rate of LDL oxidation [72b], indicating that superoxide output is not a limiting factor in these cultures. The discrepancies between these and the above studies may reflect changes in monocyte pro-oxidant mechanisms as these cells differentiate into macrophages, differences in the contribution of the medium components and/or the nature(s) of the oxidized species detected using different analytical methods. For example, direct comparison of TBARS and h.p.l.c. (with chemiluminescence detection of peroxides) measurements of monocyte-derived macrophage-mediated LDL peroxidation indicated that these methods are measuring quite different parameters of oxidation, both qualitatively and quantitatively [72b]. A similar discrepancy between TBARS and direct peroxide determination has also been shown for PMA-stimulated neutrophils [73]. In this instance, TBARS measurements indicated a five-fold increase in LDL oxidation products after PMA-stimulation of the cells, whereas cholesteryl linoleate hydroperoxide levels were not significantly increased. However, Stocker *et al.* [74] have directly demonstrated oxidation of LDL in phosphate-buffered saline (PBS) in the presence of neutrophils stimulated with PMA. Although the amounts of peroxides generated were very small, and would not be detected by more conventional assays such as TBARS, there was a clear PMA-specific increment in LDL peroxide formation in the presence of neutrophils.

In summary, the contribution of the superoxide radical in cell-mediated LDL oxidation is yet to be established. At most, it appears that any contribution of this pathway will vary considerably between cell types and the conditions under which LDL oxidation is monitored.

Reduced thiols

Thiol (R–SH) compounds can reduce transition metals:

$$R-SH + Cu^{2+} \rightarrow RS^{\cdot} + Cu^{+} + H^{+} \tag{7}$$

In the presence of oxygen, a range of radical species including superoxide, hydroxyl and thiyl (RS˙) radicals are generated. Some of these radicals are capable of initiating lipid peroxidation, while the reduced metal can propagate the process [reactions (2–5)]. Parthasarathy [75] demonstrated that cell-free oxidation of LDL in transition metal-containing media was accelerated in the presence of millimolar concentrations of reduced thiols, but that blocked or oxidized thiol compounds were ineffective. Fig. 1 illustrates how the generation of high-uptake LDL (an indirect measure of oxidation) in cell-free Ham's

Fig. 1   The cell-free modification of LDL in Ham's F-10 containing increasing concentrations of L-cysteine

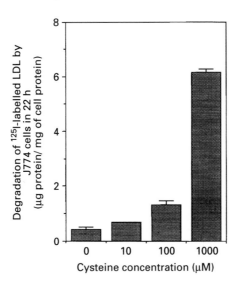

^{125}I-Labelled LDL (100 μg/ml) was incubated at 37°C for 18 h in Ham's F-10, specially formulated to be free of cysteine. The medium contained a total of 6 μM $FeSO_4$ and the indicated concentrations of freshly added L-cysteine. The LDL was then diluted to 10 μg protein/ml in serum-containing medium and its rate of degradation following uptake by mouse peritoneal macrophages measured [97]. Each histobar represents the mean ± SEM of triplicate wells of macrophages (D.J. Lamb and D.S. Leake, unpublished work).

F-10 is accelerated by increasing the concentration of L-cysteine. Heinecke et al. [76] showed that smooth muscle cell-mediated oxidation of LDL was dependent on the presence of cystine in the culture medium and suggested that the cells actively reduced the disulphide, releasing reduced thiols into the medium which, in the presence of transition metals, led to superoxide radical generation. The concomitant LDL oxidation was attributed to the activity of superoxide radical on the basis of the sensitivity of the process to added SOD, although this may have been inhibited by metal chelation rather than dismutation of superoxide (see above). More recently, the thiol-dependence of cell-mediated oxidation has been re-examined [77]. In Ham's F-10 medium supplemented with cysteine, cell-free oxidation proceeded as, or more efficiently than, endothelial cell-mediated oxidation, while in cystine-containing medium oxidation was significantly more extensive in the presence of cells (endothelial cells or macrophages). Like Heinecke 6 years previously, Sparrow and Olszewski [77] suggested that the cells were active in reduction of cystine, and indicated that this process occurred intracellularly and that LDL oxidation in a cell-free system could be accelerated by enzymic generation of reduced thiols.

Though cell-mediated reduction of cystine clearly greatly stimulates LDL oxidation in transition metal-containing media, some oxidation can still occur in the absence of added thiols [77]. Cell-mediated LDL oxidation can also be measured in a simple transition metal-containing inorganic buffer [43] (L. Kritharides, W. Jessup and R.T. Dean, unpublished work). It remains to be determined whether these processes are also associated with the secretion of reduced thiols by the cells.

Hydrogen peroxide

Hydrogen peroxide is produced by spontaneous dismutation whenever superoxide radical is generated. In the absence of transition metals it has little effect [71], but when copper is added LDL peroxidation is enhanced [78]. Catalase is reported to have no effect on the progress of cell-mediated oxidation [23,27,50,79], although others have found that catalase (even after dialysing it) can inhibit [71a]. Here it is worth noting that Steinbrecher [50] showed that an inhibitory activity associated with 'thymol-free' catalase against endothelial cell-mediated oxidation was in fact due to a heat-stable, low molecular mass contaminant which could be removed by gel-filtration or dialysis. The role of hydrogen peroxide in cell-mediated oxidation is therefore not yet resolved.

Hypochlorite

Hypochlorite (OCl^-) is produced by the myeloperoxidase of monocytes, neutrophils and eosinophils. It is a very strong oxidant which can react with lipids and proteins, e.g. by addition to double bonds to form chlorohydrins and by direct chlorination of thiol and amino groups. Treatment of LDL with reagent NaOCl *in vitro* causes immediate and preferential oxidation of the amino acids of apo B [80]. Lysine residues comprise quantitatively the major target, leading to an increase in electrophoretic mobility of the particle and its transformation to a high-uptake form which produces cholesteryl ester accumulation in macrophages. Lipid-soluble antioxidants provide little protection against this oxidative modification of LDL and only very low levels of lipid peroxides were detected. Recent work indicates that purified myeloperoxidase, together with hydrogen peroxide, produces similar changes in LDL [80a]. Though the physiological relevance of this pathway remains to be investigated, it is a potential mechanism for the oxidative transformation of LDL to a high-uptake form by newly arrived intimal monocytes, by a route which is not dependent on trace amounts of transition metals and which leaves the lipid core of the particle essentially intact. The report of normal oxidation of LDL by monocytes from a myeloperoxidase-deficient patient [36] suggests that this enzyme may not be essential in a metal-dependent oxidation system, but more extensive studies involving more patients are necessary to confirm this observation.

Reactive nitrogen species

Many of the cells of the normal and atherosclerotic intima can synthesize nitric oxide radical (NO') [81]. Nitric oxide synthase (NOS), which catalyses the conversion of L-arginine to NO and citrulline, is present constitutively in endothelial cells, where it is the vascular source of endothelial-derived relaxing factor (NO' itself or a derivative). In addition, *de novo* induction of NOS synthesis in macrophages and smooth muscle cells stimulated by inflammatory cytokines, leads to large and sustained production of NO' which is apparently only limited by substrate availability.

The nitric oxide radical is a weak reducing agent, so that LDL incubated with NO' *in vitro* does not undergo significant oxidation [82]. However, NO' can react with the superoxide radical to form peroxynitrite anion (ONOO⁻), a strong oxidant with a reactivity similar to the hydroxyl radical [83]. Treatment of LDL with 3-morpholino-synonimine-hydrochloride (SIN-1), which decomposes spontaneously to release equimolar amounts of NO' and superoxide radical, leads to extensive antioxidant consumption, lipid peroxidation [82] and (at sufficiently high molar ratios) enhanced electrophoretic mobility [84]. Authentic peroxynitrite also oxidizes LDL *in vitro*, generating an oxidized high-uptake particle [85].

Since peroxynitrite formation by PMA-stimulated rodent (rat) macrophages has been reported [86], can this oxidant contribute to cell-mediated oxidation? Paradoxically, treatment of murine macrophages with γ-interferon plus lipopolysaccharide or tumour necrosis factor-α (TNF-α) to induce NOS produces a profound suppression of their ability to oxidize LDL (Fig. 2) [82,87]. This relationship between induction of NOS activity and inhibition of LDL oxidation was confirmed when treatment of cytokine-induced macrophages with NOS inhibitors (N^G-monomethyl-L-arginine and diphenylene

Fig. 2   **Relationships between the generation of superoxide and nitric oxide radicals and cell-mediated modification of LDL by cultured macrophages**

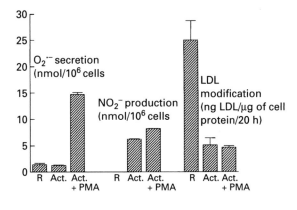

Resident peritoneal macrophages were incubated for 24 h in RPMI-1640 containing 10% (v/v) heat-inactivated fetal calf serum in the absence (R) or presence (Act.) of recombinant murine γ-interferon (100 U/ml). The media were then removed and the cells washed twice with PBS and incubated for a further 24 h in Ham's F-10 medium containing ^{125}I-LDL (100 μg protein/ml). Cell-free control incubations were performed in parallel. Nitric oxide synthesis was assayed by measurement of nitrite secretion [39] during the incubation with LDL. LDL modification was determined by measurement of ^{125}I-LDL uptake in fresh unstimulated macrophage cultures [7]. Superoxide secretion was measured during the first 90 min after addition of PMA (by which time the respiratory burst is virtually complete). Reproduced from [89] with permission.

iodonium) or incubation in arginine-free media restored their ability to oxidize LDL [39]. Exposure of resident macrophages (i.e. not induced to synthesize NO˙) to N^G-monomethyl-L-arginine had no effect on their ability to oxidize LDL [39,61,82]. Similarly, NOS inhibitors do not prevent LDL oxidation mediated by endothelial cells ([88]; W. Jessup, unpublished work). Even more interesting is the fact that PMA-stimulation of superoxide release by NO˙$^-$ secreting macrophages does not reverse the protective effect of NO˙ synthesis (Fig. 2) [82,89], suggesting that in these circumstances peroxynitrite may not be generated, at least in the vicinity of the lipoprotein particle, or that the peroxynitrite produced preferentially reaches targets other than LDL.

The basis for the protective effect of NO˙ synthesis in murine macrophage-mediated oxidation is presently under investigation. Since NO˙ forms stable chelates with free and protein-bound iron, it could prevent redox-cycling of transition metals in the cells or medium, or inhibit cellular iron-dependent enzymes such as lipoxygenases, guanylate cyclase and mito-chondrial electron transport haem proteins. Other potential targets are free and protein-bound thiols and amines, sites at which relatively stable nitrosyla-tion can occur. Ironically, the elucidation of the basis of this NO˙-dependent suppression of LDL oxidation may eventually lead us to a better understand-ing of the true mechanisms by which cells oxidize LDL *in vitro* and, hopefully, *in vivo*.

Recently γ-interferon treatment of human monocyte-macrophages has been found to suppress their ability to oxidize LDL. In this instance, reactive nitrogen species do not appear to be involved, but rather the forma-tion of antioxidant metabolites from tryptophan degradation [89a]. However, nitric oxide synthase is present in human atheroma [89b] and peroxynitrite-modified apo B has been identified in human lesions [89c].

Antioxidants and cell-mediated lipoprotein oxidation

The mechanisms by which lipid and water-soluble antioxidants prevent lipoprotein oxidation *in vitro* have been the subject of numerous reviews and are covered elsewhere in this book (see Chapter 3 by Esterbauer, this vol-ume). Here we will consider only the role of antioxidants in cell-mediated lipoprotein oxidation.

LDL contains a number of lipid-soluble antioxidants of which α-tocopherol is quantitatively the major component. During the early stages of macrophage-mediated oxidation of LDL, α-tocopherol levels declined rapidly [7] so that, after 2–4 h exposure to cells, the particles were completely depleted of this antioxidant. Since there was no detectable transfer of α-toco-pherol to the cells it was assumed that its loss was the consequence of a greater oxidative stress experienced in the presence of cells. Though loading of LDL *in vivo* by oral α-tocopherol supplementation made the lipoprotein more resistant to macrophage-mediated oxidation, no correlation has been found between the levels of α-tocopherol in non-supplemented humans and the sensitivity of the lipoprotein to cell-mediated [7,90] (or cell-free) oxidation. This suggests the presence of other quantitatively major factors influencing the progress of LDL oxidation. The system becomes more complex when it is considered that the molecular action of α-tocopherol is not simply that of a chain-breaking antioxidant, e.g. under some circumstances tocopherol may also act as a pro-oxidant [44,91]. Ubiquinol-10 is also a normal endogenous lipid-soluble antioxidant component of LDL [74]. Dietary supplementation with ubiquinone-10 leads to enrichment of LDL with the reduced, antioxidant form of the molecule (ubiquinol-10) and a corresponding increase in the resis-tance of the particle to oxidation [92].

The addition of lipid-soluble antioxidants, such as α-tocopherol [2,23,33,41,88], β-carotene [93] butylated hydroxytoluene [23,58] and probucol

[41,94], to medium supernatants during cell-mediated oxidation of LDL is surprisingly effective in inhibiting the process, since, in general, these compounds do not partition well into LDL when added in the absence of serum [95] (W. Jessup, unpublished work). Evidence has been obtained using diglutaryl probucol, which is hydrolysed intracellularly to form the active antioxidant, that part of the effect of probucol may be exerted within the modifying cells as well as extracellularly [96]. Perhaps other lipid soluble antioxidants also act directly on the modifying cells to some degree. Ascorbate protects LDL against oxidation by human monocyte-derived macrophages [34] or mouse peritoneal macrophages [96a] in the presence of transition metals and against PBMC-mediated oxidation in their absence [4], possibly by promoting tocopherol regeneration. Ascorbate can promote LDL oxidation, however, if the LDL is already partially oxidized, both in the presence or absence of cells [96a].

A large number of compounds have now been shown to inhibit LDL oxidation but the likely physiological or pharmacological importance of many of these remains to be evaluated. These include dietary components, such as flavonoids, which are consumed in the normal human diet at about 25 mg to 1 g per day and inhibit macrophage-mediated LDL oxidation by 50% at concentrations of 1–20 μM [97,98]. The flavonoids conserve the α-tocopherol content of LDL and delay the onset of lipid peroxidation [97]. Whether or not flavonoids are a naturally occurring anti-atherogenic component of the diet will, however, depend very much on their pharmacokinetics, and very little is known of this in man. High concentrations (100 μM) of two particular flavonoids, myricetin and gossypetin, induce non-oxidative cross-linking and aggregation of LDL, which lead to its greatly increased scavenger receptor-independent uptake by macrophages [99]. However, it is unlikely that these concentrations would be achieved *in vivo*. A number of other naturally occurring antioxidants inhibit LDL oxidation by copper and may possibly function protectively *in vivo*; these include phenolic compounds present in China green tea [100], Japanese herbal Kampo medicines [101] and red wine [102], and the hormone α-oestradiol [103]. Zinc inhibits LDL oxidation by macrophages [103a].

Cell-mediated LDL oxidation can be inhibited by a number of drugs used in clinical medicine or under trial. Several of these drugs also prevent cell-free copper oxidation of LDL. These include the antihypertensives carvedilol [104], indapamide [105], several calcium antagonists (ryanodine, nifedipine, verapamil, flunarizine) [106], cholesterol synthesis inhibitors simvastatin and lovastatin [107,108], aminoguanidine [109], a 21-aminosteroid [110] and phenothiazines (e.g. chlorpromazine) [111]. LDL isolated from patients given the lipid-lowering drugs pravastatin, bezafibrate or cholestyramine has been found to be less susceptible to copper or cell-mediated oxidation, although pravastatin and bezafibrate had no antioxidant effect *in vitro*. High concentrations of the β-blockers, propranolol, pindolol and metoprolol, decreased LDL oxidation by endothelial cells [112]; the anti-inflammatory compound, leumedin, inhibited mild oxidation of LDL in a coculture system containing endothelial and smooth muscle cells [113] by an unknown mechanism.

Serum is a very good inhibitor of LDL oxidation by cells [4,41,58,114]. Significant LDL oxidation is therefore unlikely to occur in the circulation. The relative order of antioxidant protection by individual components of plasma has not been detailed, but some inhibitory components have been identified. HDL spares LDL oxidized by cells or copper, probably at least in part by providing an alternative oxidizable substrate [5,18], and because it contains the enzyme paraoxonase [115], and in doing so it suppresses the formation of high-uptake LDL (Fig. 3). Lipoprotein-deficient

Fig. 3   Inhibition by HDL of LDL modification by macrophages

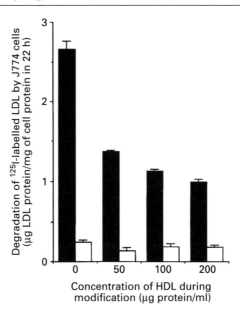

Concentration of HDL during
modification (μg protein/ml)

Human ^{125}I-labelled LDL (100 μg protein/ml) was incubated for 20 h with mouse resident peritoneal macrophages (macrophage-modified LDL; black histobars) or cell-free wells (control LDL; white histobars) in the presence of unlabelled human HDL (up to 200 μg protein/ml). It was then diluted 1 in 10 in serum-containing medium and incubated for 22 h with J774 macrophage-like cells and its degradation by them measured as an indication of its rate of uptake. Each histobar represents the mean ± SEM of triplicate wells of peritoneal macrophages. (G.M. Wilkins and D.S. Leake, unpublished work).

serum (dialysed and therefore lacking water-soluble antioxidants such as ascorbate) also inhibits effectively [50], of which a major protective component is almost certainly albumin, probably by virtue of its metal-chelating properties [72a] as well as acting as a sacrificial substrate to the highly reactive oxidants produced in the presence of transition metals.

Oxidized lipoproteins and cell function

Metabolism of oLDL by macrophages

Although the endocytosis of oxidized and acetylated LDL by macrophages is mediated largely (though not necessarily exclusively [116]) by common receptors, and both occur rapidly, there are marked differences in the intracellular fates of these lipoproteins. In fact, most studies on this topic have addressed the fate of the apolipoprotein component of oLDL; relatively less is known of the metabolism of oLDL-derived lipids.

A number of studies have indicated that cells cultured with oLDL progressively accumulate macromolecular deposits of apo B. In general, during a 24 h period of uptake, endocytosed acetylated LDL apo B is rapidly degraded (>90%) to low molecular mass products released into the medium, whereas up to 50% of the apo B of endocytosed oLDL is retained within the cells as high molecular mass (TCA-insoluble) material [117–122]. The amount of apo B which accumulates intracellularly is related to the degree to which it has been oxidized [120,121] and this residual pool of undegraded intracellular material is particularly resistant to further degradation ($t_{0.5} \sim 48$ h) during a subsequent chase period [121]. It is now clear that the reason for the impaired degradation of the apo B of oLDL within macrophages is its intrinsic resistance to lysosomal proteolysis. This is based on the following observations; (i) oLDL is resistant to degradation by macrophage acid proteases [117,121,122] and to purified lysosomal cathepsins; (ii) endocytosed oLDL colocalizes with lysosomal but not endosomal markers detected by immunofluorescence microscopy [122a] and (iii) subcellular fractionation indicates that ^{125}I-labelled, TCA-insoluble material accumulates in the lysosomal compartment after incubation of cells with ^{125}I-oLDL (Fig. 4). Interestingly, this accumulation does not appear to influence the rates of endocytosis and degradation of other lipoproteins [120,122,123] or of ligands for other receptors [121,122].

The reason for the resistance of oxidized apo B to lysosomal proteolysis is not yet completely understood. It may be the consequence of covalent modifications to this protein by lipid peroxidation products [120,121], by formation of novel stable protein–protein cross-links [71,121], by the introduction of novel amino acid modifications [124], by the inactivation of cathepsin B [124a], or by a combination of all of these. We have recently

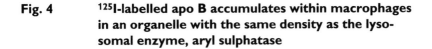

Fig. 4   **^{125}I-labelled apo B accumulates within macrophages in an organelle with the same density as the lysosomal enzyme, aryl sulphatase**

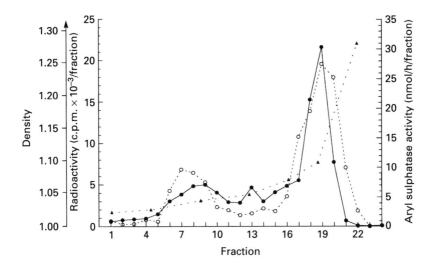

J774 macrophages were incubated with ^{125}I-labelled copper-oxidized LDL for 60 min, washed, homogenized and the post-nuclear supernatant fractionated on an isotonic 1–22% Ficoll gradient underlaid with a 45% Nycodenz cushion. Individual fractions were assayed for radioactivity (●), aryl sulphatase activity (○), and the refractive index was used to calculate density (▲). Reproduced from [122a] with permission.

shown that a component of oxidized bovine serum albumin is also resistant to lysosomal proteolysis and accumulates within macrophages following endocytic uptake [125], indicating that the phenomenon is not restricted to lipoproteins.

It is not surprising that oLDL is less efficient than acetylated LDL in promoting cholesterol accumulation in macrophages, because oxidation leads to a substantial depletion of cholesteryl esters and (to a lesser degree) cholesterol in the lipoprotein as they are converted to a range of oxidized esters and oxysterols, of which the most abundant are 7-ketocholesterol and 7-hydroxycholesterol [9a,119]. In addition, the observed stimulation of cholesterol esterification in macrophages by oLDL is approximately half that obtained with acetylated LDL, even after correcting for the amount of cholesterol delivered to the cells. These effects can be accounted for if the combined effects of the lower cholesterol content together with the slower rate of cellular degradation of oLDL are calculated [119]. This observation raises the possibility that lysosomal degradation of the whole oxidized lipoprotein particle is inhibited, and suggests that there is an interdependence between degradation of the lipid and protein components. A prediction which would follow from this is that a substantial proportion of the lipid which accumulates in macrophages loaded with oLDL will be located initially within the lysosomes. It is possible that the ceroid deposits which are found both in macrophages cultured with oLDL [126] and in atheromatous lesions *in vivo* [126a] are derived at least partly from endocytosis of oxidized, and thus intrinsically indigestible, lipoproteins.

The oxysterols present in oLDL taken up by cells may affect the intracellular processing of the particle. For example, Zhang *et al.* [119] found that of a range of oxysterols present in oLDL, tested individually for their effects on cholesterol esterification, both stimulatory and inhibitory components were identified. 7-Ketocholesterol, an abundant oxysterol in oLDL, was stimulatory when added directly as a solution. However, it is less certain whether delivery of such molecules as integral components of lipoproteins will give them access to the same range of intracellular targets.

We have recently found that the normal pathways used by cells to remove cholesterol (reverse cholesterol transport) are much less efficient at removing cholesterol, particularly 7-ketocholesterol, from cells which accumulate oLDL [125a]. When exposed to extracellular apo AI for 24 h, acetylated LDL-derived foam cells released 50% of their total cholesterol content (as free cholesterol), whereas oLDL-loaded cells exported only 30% of total cellular cholesterol and 7% of their 7-ketocholesterol content (Fig. 5). We do not yet know whether this is a consequence of the intracellular location of the lipid deposits and their accessibility to reverse cholesterol transport or of an inhibitory activity of oxidized products such as 7-ketocholesterol on the process.

Cellular effects of oLDL

The composition of LDL changes continuously as it undergoes oxidation [12], even after other parameters such as its electrophoretic mobility and TBARS content have reached their maximum. Several of the individual, and often transient, oxidation products have been identified as active modulators of cell functions. However, in most cases the degree to which LDL has been oxidized is not well-defined and the active component(s) have not been identified. Almost without exception, the studies described below have been performed using copper-oxidized LDL; it is assumed that since the same major oxidation products are generated in cell-oxidized LDL, this will have similar biological activities.

oLDL is directly chemotactic for human monocytes, in part due to

Fig. 5   Reverse cholesterol transport from foam cells loaded with acetylated or oxidized LDL

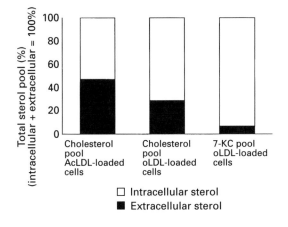

Murine peritoneal macrophages were incubated for 24 h in DMEM with 10% (v/v) heat-inactivated fetal calf serum containing acetylated LDL (50 μg protein/ml; AcLDL-loaded cells) or copper-oxidized LDL (50 μg protein/ml; oLDL-loaded cells). The cells were then incubated for a further 24 h in DMEM containing apo AI (25 μg/ml) and albumin (100 μg/ml). The efflux of cholesterol and (for oLDL-loaded cells) 7-ketocholesterol (7-KC) into the supernatants was measured by h.p.l.c. [12]. The 100% (intracellular plus released) values were: AcLDL loaded cells, 250 nmol (cholesterol plus cholesteryl esters)/mg cell protein; oLDL-loaded cells, 175 nmol (cholesterol+cholesteryl esters)/mg cell protein; 30 nmol 7-keto-cholesterol/mg LDL protein. Cells contain both free and esterified cholesterol, but only free cholesterol is released. No significant efflux occurs in the absence of apo AI. Reproduced from [125a] with permission.

its lysophosphatidylcholine content [127], and may thus be involved in recruiting monocytes into atherosclerotic lesions. Lysophosphatidylcholine is not chemotactic for neutrophils, which may be of significance as atherosclerotic lesions contain very few of these cells, but it is chemotactic for smooth muscle cells [128], which may influence their migration from the media to the intima in atherosclerotic lesions. The migration of endothelial cells, on the other hand, is inhibited by oLDL [129]. In contrast to its effects on monocytes, oLDL decreases the motility of macrophages (the cells which monocytes differentiate into in the tissues) and may thus serve to trap these cells in the arterial wall [127]. It has been shown that oLDL induces the adhesion of leucocytes to arterioles and venules *in vivo* in hamsters, apparently by a superoxide- and leukotriene-dependent process [130]. It also induces the differentiation of monocytes and their adhesion to endothelial cells [131], indicating that local differentiation of monocytes in atherosclerotic lesions may be accelerated in the presence of oLDL. The proliferation of mouse peritoneal macrophages in culture is stimulated by oxidized but not native LDL [132], which may explain why macrophages apparently divide in atherosclerotic lesions [133].

It has been known for some time that oLDL is toxic to cells [134]; recently its toxicity to macrophages has been demonstrated [135]. oLDL initially decreases and later increases the intracellular glutathione content of macrophages [136], which may be relevant in its toxicity. Macrophage death is a prominent feature of advanced lesions in humans and is possibly an important factor in the progression of these lesions [135].

oLDL has been reported to induce changes in a number of intracellular and secreted metabolites. These include potential stimulation of thrombus formation by increased platelet aggregation [137], increased secretion of plasminogen activator inhibitor-1 from endothelial cells [138] and expression of tissue factor activity by endothelial cells [139] and a decrease of their protein C activation (activated protein C inactivates Factors Va and VIIIa) [140]. Intracellular free calcium can also be increased by oLDL in vascular smooth muscle cells [141] and endothelial cells [142]. It has also been reported to either stimulate [143] or inhibit [144] phosphoinositide turnover in endothelial cells and to increase it in smooth muscle cells [145]. Prostaglandin and leukotriene synthesis by macrophages can be increased by oLDL [146] but it can also be decreased if the cells are pre-incubated with oLDL [147]. Prostaglandin synthesis by smooth muscle cells has been shown to be decreased by oLDL [148]. These discrepancies may arise from differences in the composition of individual oLDL preparations as well as the exact conditions of the experiments. The rate of fluid-phase pinocytosis by cultured endothelial cells was reduced by oLDL, apparently before any toxic effect occurred [149].

Platelet-derived growth factor release by endothelial cells [150] or macrophages [151] is reduced by oLDL, but is increased in smooth muscle cells [152]. The effect on smooth muscle cells may help to explain why these cells proliferate in lesions; the effect on macrophages is of interest because about 20% of macrophages in atherosclerotic lesions contain this growth factor, but the levels in macrophage-derived foam cells are very low [153]. oLDL also suppresses TNF-α expression in macrophages [154] but increases their release of interleukin-1β (which stimulates smooth muscle cell proliferation) [29,155]. oLDL is highly immunogenic and antibodies that bind to it are present in animals and in many humans [156,157]. Very low concentrations of oLDL can activate T-lymphocytes and this may be of significance, as human atherosclerotic lesions contain activated T-lymphocytes [29].

There has been much interest recently in the effects of mildly oxidized (or 'minimally modified') LDL, since its effects are very different from those of the highly oxidized LDL usually studied. Mildly oxidized LDL is produced by prolonged storage or by incubation with ferrous sulphate or, more recently, with soybean lipoxygenase and phospholipase A_2. In contrast to highly oxidized LDL, mildly oxidized LDL still binds to the apo B/E receptor and not to the scavenger receptors [11]. Also in contrast to highly oxidized LDL, mildly oxidized LDL induces the genes on endothelial cells for cellular adhesion molecules for monocytes, for monocyte chemotactic protein-1(MCP-1) [11,158], for tissue factor [159] and for various types of colony stimulating factor [160]. A remarkable feature of mildly oxidized LDL is its potency; as little as 0.05 mg protein/ml can affect the function of endothelial cells.

Fig. 6 indicates how some of these properties of oLDL may play a role in the development of atherosclerotic lesions. In many respects the early stages of the lesion resemble a type of inflammatory response. Thus, mildly oxidized LDL, if generated in the intima by the activity of local cells, may induce the expression of cellular adhesion molecules and MCP-1 synthesis by endothelial and smooth muscle cells, leading to monocyte (and possibly lymphocyte) infiltration. Within the intima, monocyte differentiation into macrophages (which express scavenger receptors) and their contribution to LDL oxidation may further promote LDL oxidation and its uptake, leading to foam cell development. It is still not clear why mildly oxidized LDL would form in particular sites (i.e. lesion-prone areas). Interestingly, NO availability is generally depressed in the hyperlipidaemic intima; perhaps this molecule normally has a protective antioxidant function *in vivo* (described above) which is compromised in conditions of hyperlipidaemia. Once lipoprotein oxidation is established, a self-reinforcing situation may occur, since oLDL appears to attenuate the availability of NO in the intima [161] and the capacity of activated cells to release further NO is decreased when they are pre-exposed to oLDL [162].

Significance of cell-mediated lipoprotein oxidation *in vivo*

The question frequently levelled at almost all *in vitro* studies of cell-mediated oxidation is, of course, 'what is their relevance to pathophysiology?' Can a process which can only be detected *in vitro* in a metal- and oxygen-enriched, antioxidant-deficient medium truly be an accurate, if accelerated, reflection of events which occur in the intima? Certainly there is ample evidence that lipid oxidation products are present in atheromatous lesions, though whether it is causal or secondary to other initiating events in lesion formation is much less

Fig. 6   Mildly oxidized LDL may be involved in the initiation of fatty streaks and highly oxidized LDL may be involved in their progression

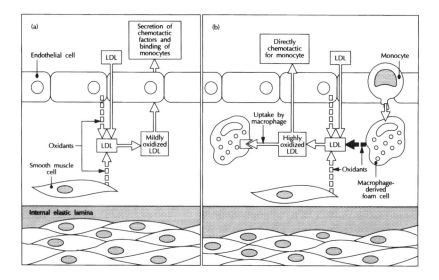

(a) LDL may enter the arterial intima, which may be very thin in animals but thicker in humans due to diffuse intimal thickening, and may then be converted into mildly oxidized LDL by free radicals or by oxidized lipids released from the endothelial or smooth muscle cells (––→). This mildly oxidized LDL may cause the endothelial cells to release greater amounts of a chemotactic factor for monocytes (and possibly lymphocytes?) and to bind the monocytes to a greater extent. (b) The monocytes may then enter the arterial intima, differentiate into macrophages, release large amounts of free radicals or oxidized lipids (■▶) and convert the LDL into highly oxidized LDL. This may bind to scavenger receptors on the macrophages, be internalized rapidly and convert them to cholesterol-laden foam cells. The highly oxidized LDL may be directly chemotactic for monocytes (due to its lysophosphatidyl-choline content) and may attract more monocytes into the arterial wall, leading to the progression of the lesions. Reproduced from [175] with permission.

clear. Thus, antioxidants do appear to retard the progression of atherosclerotic lesions, but their primary activity in the process may be at a level other than as inhibitors of lipoprotein oxidation. However, a recent study using intact vessels [163] indirectly indicates that generation of oLDL and its uptake by foam cells does occur in the intima *in vivo*, and that this can be blocked by addition of vitamin E to the system.

Recent careful examination of the product pattern of peroxidized lipids present in human atheromata gave little clue to their origins, indicating a predominantly non-enzymic route of formation [65]. Thus, even if lipoxygenases have an initiating role in lipoprotein oxidation in the intima, a non-enzymic, perhaps metal-dependent, sequence of events must follow. If metals are involved in lipoprotein oxidation, then most of the other cellular mechanisms of lipoprotein oxidation discussed above may also be participants. Although iron and copper are present in all tissues, they are normally bound to protein in a redox-inactive state. Nevertheless, some recent studies have indicated associations; (i) between serum copper levels and lesion progression [164]; (ii) between the risk of myocardial infarction and serum ferritin levels, in a prospective study [165] (although this study, surprisingly, did not adjust for antioxidant levels as independent risk factors and other studies do not agree with it) and (iii) iron and copper levels were shown to be elevated in aortic tissue from patients with occlusive and aneurysmal disease compared with controls [166]. These studies suggest that increased metal availability is associated with lesion development. Some evidence has recently been reported for the presence of catalytically active iron and copper in 'gruel' prepared from post-mortem human advanced lesions [167]. Examination of these data indicates that in fact there was no (or only very poor) correlation between the detectable 'free' iron and copper contents of these samples and their pro-oxidant activities but this may possibly be due to various antioxidants also present in the gruel.

What remains to be established is whether these changes in metal content precede lesion formation or arise as a consequence of it, and what, if any, relationship they have to intimal LDL oxidation. The source of the intimal metals is also not clear. Iron might be derived from infiltrating plasma proteins exposed to cellular oxidants, haem proteins released by damaged intimal cells in more advanced lesions and from ruptured erythrocytes in areas of haemorrhage. Haemin can catalyse LDL oxidation in the presence of peroxides, and in the process free iron is released [168]; haemoglobin will also catalyse LDL oxidation [169]. Transition metal ions bound to proteins such as transferrin and caeruloplasmin become catalytically active at low pH and can oxidize LDL [170,171]. Such regions may exist in localized areas of the intima.

As yet, relatively little attention has been given to the contribution of the surrounding tissue architecture to lipoprotein oxidation. Direct physical interactions between closely apposed cells which have large areas of mutual contact, and between cells and extracellular matrix, may influence their oxidative activity, their access to target lipoprotein particles and the extracellular pH. Diffusible mediators from surrounding cells may influence oxidative processes by more efficient or different mechanisms in 3-dimensional tissue compared with their effect measured in our simple tissue culture systems.

Extracellular matrix may be important in the retention of lipoproteins in the intima, particularly Lp(a) [172], and may even influence their sensitivity to oxidation [173]. There is clearly a need for studies of lipoprotein oxidation to move towards systems which can incorporate some of these features into their design. Some early studies with these more complex systems have already yielded interesting and exciting data on related aspects of atherogenesis [174], and offer the promise of an answer to the question posed above in the near future.

References
1.   Henriksen, T., Mahoney, E.M. and Steinberg, D. (1981) Proc. Natl. Acad. Sci. U.S.A. **78**, 6499–6503
2.   Steinbrecher, U.P., Parthasarathy, S., Leake, D.S., Witztum, J.L. and Steinberg, D. (1984) Proc. Natl. Acad. Sci. U.S.A. **81**, 3883–3887
3.   Henriksen, T., Mahoney, E.M. and Steinberg, D. (1982) Ann. N.Y. Acad. Sci. **401**, 102–116
4.   Frei, B., Stocker, R. and Ames, B.N. (1988) Proc. Natl. Acad. Sci. U.S.A. **85**, 9748–9752
5.   Bowry, V.W., Stanley, K.K. and Stocker, R. (1992) Proc. Natl. Acad. Sci. U.S.A. **89**, 10316–10320
6.   Esterbauer, H., Gebicki, J., Puhl, H. and Jurgens, G. (1992) Free Radical Biol. Med. **13**, 341–390
7.   Jessup, W., Rankin, S.M., de Whalley, C.V., Hoult, J.R.S., Scott, J. and Leake, D.S. (1990) Biochem. J. **265**, 399–405
8.   Wang, T., Yu, W.G. and Powell, W.S. (1992) J. Lipid Res. **33**, 525–537
9.   Jialal, I., Freeman, D.A. and Grundy, S.M. (1991) Arteriosclerosis Thrombosis **11**, 482–488
9a.   Carpenter, K.L.H., Wilkins, G.M., Fussell, B., Ballantine, J.A., Taylor, S.E., Mitchinson, M.J. and Leake, D.S. (1994) Biochem. J. **304**, 625–633
10.   Bhadra, S., Arshad, M.A.Q., Rymaszewski, Z., Norman, E., Wherley, R. and Subbiah, M.T.R. (1991) Biochim. Biophys. Res. Commun. **176**, 431–440
11.   Berliner, J.A., Territo, M.C., Sevanian, A., Ramin, S., Kim, J.A., Ramshad, B., Esterson, M. and Fogelman, A.M. (1990) J. Clin. Invest. **85**, 1260–1266
12.   Kritharides, L., Jessup, W., Gifford, J. and Dean, R.T. (1993) Anal. Biochem. **213**, 79–89
13.   Parthasarathy, S., Weiland, E. and Steinberg, D. (1989) Proc. Natl. Acad. Sci. U.S.A. **86**, 1046–1050
13a. Aviram, M. and Rosenblat, M. (1994) J. Lipid Res. **35**, 385–398
14.   Steinberg, D., Parthasarathy, S., Carew, T.E., Khoo, J.C. and Witztum, J.L. (1989) New Engl. J. Med. **320**, 915–924
15.   Witztum, J.L. and Steinberg, D. (1991) J. Clin. Invest. **88**, 1785–1792
16.   Parthasarathy, S. and Rankin, S.M. (1992) Prog. Lipid Res. **31**, 127–143
17.   Henriksen, T., Mahoney, E.M. and Steinberg, D. (1983) Arteriosclerosis **3**, 149–159
18.   Parthasarathy, S., Barnett, J. and Fong, L.G. (1990) Biochim. Biophys. Acta. **1044**, 275–283
19.   Parthasarathy, S., Quinn, M.T., Schwenke, D.C., Carew, T.E. and Steinberg, D. (1989) Arteriosclerosis **9**, 398–404
20.   Horrigan, S., Campbell, J.H. and Campbell, G.R. (1991) Arteriosclerosis Thrombosis **11**, 279–289
21.   Naruszewicz, M., Selinger, E. and Davignon, J. (1990) Arteriosclerosis **10**, 808a
22.   Carpenter, K.L.H., Ballantine, J.A., Fussell, B., Enright, J.H. and Mitchinson, M.J. (1990) Atherosclerosis **83**, 217–229
23.   van Hinsbergh, V.W.M., Scheffer, M., Havekes, L. and Kempen, H.J.M. (1986) Biochim. Biophys. Acta. **878**, 49–64
24.   Derian, C.K. and Lewis, D.F. (1992) Prostagland. Leukotr. Essent. Fatty Acids **45**, 49–57
25.   Morgan, J., Smith, J.A., Wilkins, G.M. and Leake, D.S. (1993) Atherosclerosis **102**, 209–216
26.   Heinecke, J.W., Rosen, H. and Chait, A. (1984) J. Clin. Invest. **74**, 1890–1894
27.   Heinecke, J.W., Rosen, H. and Chait, A. (1986) J. Clin. Invest. **77**, 757–761
28.   Lamb, D.J., Wilkins, G.M. and Leake, D.S. (1992) Atherosclerosis **92**, 187–192

29. Frostegard, J., Wu, R., Giscombe, R., Holm, G., Lefvert, A.K. and Nilsson, J. (1992) Arteriosclerosis Thrombosis **12**, 461–467
30. Lamb, D.J. and Leake, D.S. (1993) Biochem. Soc. Trans. **21**, 132S
31. Parthasarathy, S., Printz, D.J., Boyd, D., Joy, L. and Steinberg, D. (1986) Arteriosclerosis **6**, 505–510
32. Rankin, S.M. and Leake, D.S. (1987) Biochem. Soc. Trans. **15**, 485–486
33. Cathcart, M.K., Morel, D.W. and Chisolm III, G.M. (1985)J. Leukocyte Biol. **38**, 341–350
34. Jialal, I. and Grundy, S.M. (1991) J. Clin. Invest. **87**, 597–601
35. Wilkins, G.M., Segal, A.W. and Leake, D.S. (1994) Biochem. Biophys. Res. Commun. **202**, 1300–1307
36. Hiramatsu, K., Rosen, H., Heinecke, J.W., Wolfbauer, G. and Chait, A. (1987) Arteriosclerosis **7**, 55–60
36a. Wilkins, G.M. and Leake, D.S. (1994) Biochim. Biophys. Acta **1215**, 250–258
37. Rosenfeld, M.E., Khoo, J.C., Miller, E., Parthasarathy, S., Palinski, W. and Witztum, J.L. (1991) J. Clin. Invest. **87**, 90–99
38. Gorog, P. and Kakkar, V.V. (1987) Atherosclerosis **65**, 99–107
39. Jessup, W. and Dean, R.T. (1993) Atherosclerosis **101**, 145–155
40. Steinbrecher, U.P., Witztum, J.L., Parthasarathy, S. and Steinberg, D. (1987) Arteriosclerosis **7**, 135–143
41. Leake, D.S. and Rankin, S.M. (1990) Biochem. J. **270**, 741–748
41a. Lamb, D.J., Hider, R.C. and Leake, D.S. (1993) Biochem. Soc. Trans. **21**, 234S
42. Cathcart, M.K., Chisolm, G.M., McNally, A.K. and Morel, D.W. (1988) In Vitro Cell. Dev. **24**, 1001–1008
43. Morgan, J. and Leake, D.S. (1993) FEBS Lett. **333**, 275–279
44. Bowry, V.W. and Stocker, R. (1993) J. Am. Chem. Soc. **115**, 6029–6044
45. Thomas, C.E. and Jackson, R.L. (1991) J. Pharmacol. Exp. Ther. **256**, 1182–1188
46. Dunford, H.B. (1987) Free Radical Biol. Med. **3**, 405–421
47. Jessup, W., Simpson, J.A. and Dean, R.T. (1993) Atherosclerosis **101**, 107–120
48. Cathcart, M.K., McNally, A.K., Morel, D.W. and Chisolm, G.M. (1989) J. Immunol. **142**, 1963–1969
49. Buettner, G.R. (1988) J. Biochem. Biophys. Methods **16**, 27–33
50. Steinbrecher, U.P. (1988) Biochim. Biophys. Acta. **959**, 20–30
51. Sparrow, C.P., Parthasarathy, S. and Steinberg, D. (1988) J. Lipid Res. **29**, 745–753
52. McNally, A.K., Chisolm, G.M., Morel, D.W. and Cathcart, M.K. (1990) J. Immunol. **145**, 254–259
53. Rankin, S.M., Parthasarathy, S. and Steinberg, D. (1991) J. Lipid Res. **32**, 449–456
54. Pace-Asciak, C.R. and Asotra, S. (1989) Free Radical Biol. Med. **7**, 409–433
55. Kuhn, H., Belkner, J., Wiesner, R. and Brash, A. (1991)J. Biol. Chem. **65**, 18351–18361
56. Belkner, J., Wiesner, R., Rathman, J., Barnett, J., Sigal, E. and Kuhn, H. (1993) Eur. J. Biochem. **213**, 251–261
57. O'Leary, V.J., Darley-Usmar, V.M., Russell, L.J. and Stone, D. (1992) Biochem. J. **282**, 631–634
58. Jessup, W., Darley-Usmar, V.M., O'Leary, V. and Bedwell, S. (1991) Biochem. J. **278**, 163–169
59. Folcik, V.A. and Cathcart, M.K. (1993) J. Lipid Res. **34**, 69–79
60. Sparrow, C.P. and Olszewski, J. (1992) Proc. Natl. Acad. Sci. U.S.A. **89**, 128–131
61. Wilkins, G.M. and Leake, D.S. (1994) Biochim. Biophys. Acta. **1211**, 69–78
62. Wilkins, G.M. and Leake, D.S. (1990) Biochem. Soc. Trans. **18**, 1170–1171
63. Henricksson, P., Hamberg, M. and Dicfalusy, U. (1985) Biochim. Biophys. Acta. **834**, 272–274
64. Yla-Herttuala, S., Rosenfeld, M.E., Parthasarathy, S., Glass, C.K., Sigal, E., Witztum, J.L. and Steinberg, D. (1990) Proc. Natl. Acad. Sci. U.S.A. **87**, 6959–6963
65. Kuhn, H., Belkner, J., Wiesner, R., Schewe, T., Lankin, V.Z. and Tikhaze, A.K. (1992) Eicosanoids **5**, 17–22
65a. Kuhn, H., Belkner, J., Zaiss, S., Fahrenklemper, T. and Wohlfeil, S. (1994) J. Exp. Med. **179**, 1903–1911
66. Thomas, J.P., Geiger, P.G., Maiorino, M., Ursini, F. and Girotti, A.W. (1990) Biochim. Biophys. Acta. **1045**, 252–260

67. Simon, T.C., Makheja, A.N. and Bailey, J.M. (1989) Atherosclerosis **75**, 31–38
68. Simon, T.C., Makheja, A.N. and Bailey, J.M. (1989) Thromb. Res. **55**, 171–178
68a. Mol, M.J.T.M., Benz, D., Mori-Ito, N., Ezaki, M., Parthasarathy, S., Steinberg, D. and Witztum, J.L. (1994) Atherosclerosis **109**, 40
68b. Myllyharju, H., Kaunismaki, T., Laukkanen, M., Nikkari, T. and Yla-Herttuala, S. (1994) Atherosclerosis **109**, 107
69. Steinbrecher, U.P., Zhang, H. and Lougheed, M. (1990) Free Radical Biol. Med. **9**, 155–168
70. Gebicki, J.M. and Bielski, B.J.H. (1981) J. Am. Chem. Soc. **103**, 7020–7022
71. Bedwell, S., Dean, R.T. and Jessup, W. (1989) Biochem. J. **262**, 707–712
71a. Wilkins, G.M. and Leake, D.S. (1994) Biochim. Biophys. Acta **1215**, 250–258
72. Morel, D.W., Hessler, J.R. and Chisolm, G.M. (1983) J. Lipid Res. **24**, 1070–1076
72a. Thomas, C.E. (1992) Biochim. Biophys. Acta. **1128**, 50–57
72b. Garner, B., Dean, R.T. and Jessup, W. (1994) Biochem. J. **301**, 421–428
73. Abdalla, D.S., Campa, A. and Monteiro, H.P. (1992) Atherosclerosis **97**, 149–159
74. Stocker, R., Bowry, V.W. and Frei, B. (1991) Proc. Natl. Acad. Sci. U.S.A. **88**, 1646–1650
75. Parthasarathy, S. (1987) Biochim. Biophys. Acta. **917**, 337–340
76. Heinecke, J.W., Rosen, H., Suzuki, L.A. and Chait, A. (1987) J. Biol. Chem. **262**, 10098–10103
77. Sparrow, C. and Olszewski, C.P. (1993) J. Lipid Res. **34**, 1219–1228
78. Montgomery, R.R., Nathan, C.F. and Cohn, Z.A. (1986) Proc. Natl. Acad. Sci. U.S.A. **83**, 6631–6635
79. Hessler, J.R., Morel, D.W., Lewis, J. and Chisolm, G.M. (1983) Arteriosclerosis **3**, 215–222
80. Hazell, L. and Stocker, R. (1993) Biochem. J. **290**, 165–172
80a. Hazell, L.J., van den Berg, J.J.M. and Stocker, R. (1994) Biochem. J. **302**, 297–304
81. Nathan, C. (1992) FASEB J. **6**, 3051–3604
82. Jessup, W., Mohr, D., Gieseg, S.P., Dean, R.T. and Stocker, R. (1992) Biochim. Biophys. Acta. **1180**, 73–82
83. Beckman, J.S., Beckman, T.W., Chen, J., Marshall, P.A. and Freeman, B.A. (1990) Proc. Natl. Acad. Sci. U.S.A. **87**, 1620–1624
84. Darley-Usmar, V.M., Hogg, N., O'Leary, V.J., Wilson, M.T. and Moncada, S. (1992) Free Radical Res. Commun. **17**, 9–20
85. Hogg, N., Darley-Usmar, V.M., Graham, A. and Moncada, S. (1993) Biochem. Soc. Trans. **21**, 358–362
86. Ischiropoulos, H., Zhu, L. and Beckman, J.S. (1992) Arch. Biochem. Biophys. **298**, 446–451
87. Yates, M.T., Lambert, L.E., Whitten, J.P., McDonald, I., Mano, M., Ku, G. and Mao, S.J.T. (1992) FEBS Lett. **309**, 135–138
88. Morgan, J., Smith, J.A., Wilkins, G.M. and Leake, D.S. (1993) Atherosclerosis **102**, 209–216
89. Jessup, W. (1993) Biochem. Soc. Trans. **21**, 321–325
89a. Christen, S., Thomas, S.R., Garner, B. and Stocker, R. (1994) J. Clin. Invest. **93**, 2149–2158
89b. Luoma, J., Sarkioja, T., Nikkari, T. and Yla-Herttuala, S. (1994) Atherosclerosis **109**, 102
89c. Beckman, J.S., Ye, Y.Z., Anderson, P.G., Chen, J., Accavitti, M.A., Tarpey, M.M. and White, C.R. (1994) Biol. Chem. Hoppe Seyler **375**, 81–88
90. Reaven, P.D., Khouw, A., Beltz, W.F., Parthasarathy, S. and Witztum, J.L. (1993) Arteriosclerosis Thrombosis **13**, 590–600
91. Bowry, V.W., Ingold, K.U. and Stocker, R. (1992) Biochem J. **288**, 341–344
92. Mohr, D., Bowry, V.W. and Stocker, R. (1992) Biochim. Biophys. Acta. **1126**, 247–254
93. Jialal, I., Norkus, E.P., Cristol, L. and Grundy, S.M. (1991) Biochim. Biophys. Acta. **1086**, 134–138
94. Parthasarathy, S., Young, S.G., Witztum, J.L., Pittman, R.C. and Steinberg, D. (1986) J. Clin. Invest. **77**, 641–644
95. Esterbauer, H., Puhl, H., Dieber, R.M., Waeg, G. and Rabl, H. (1991) Ann. Med. **23**, 573–581
96. Parthasarathy, S. (1992) J. Clin. Invest. **89**, 1618–1621
96a. Stait, S.E. and Leake, D.S. (1994) FEBS Lett. **341**, 263–267
97. de Whalley, C.V., Rankin, S.M., Hoult, J.R.S., Jessup, W. and Leake, D.S. (1990) Biochem. Pharmacol. **39**, 1743–1750
98. Mangiapane, H., Thomson, J., Salter, A., Brown, S., Bell, G.D. and White, D.A. (1992) Biochem. Pharmacol. **43**, 445–450

99. Rankin, S.M., de Whalley, C.V., Hoult, J.R.S., Jessup, W., Wilkins, G.M., Collard, J. and Leake, D.S. (1993) Biochem. Pharmacol. **45**, 67–75
100. Zhenhua, D., Yuan, C., Mei, Z. and Yunzhong, F. (1991) Med. Sci. Res. **19**, 767–768
101. Ondrias, K., Stasko, A., Gergel, D., Hromadova, M. and Benes, L. (1992) Free Radical Res. Commun. **16**, 227–237
102. Frankel, E.N., Kanner, J., German, J.B., Parks, E. and Kinsella, J.E. (1993) Lancet **341**, 454–457
103. Maziere, C., Auclair, M., Ronveaux, M.F., Salmon, S., Santus, R. and Maziere, J.C. (1991) Atherosclerosis **89**, 175–182
103a. Wilkins, G.M. and Leake, D.S. (1994) FEBS Lett. **341**, 259–262
104. Yue, T.L., McKenna, P.J., Lysko, P.G., Ruffolo, R.J. and Feuerstein, G.Z. (1992) Atherosclerosis **97**, 209–216
105. Breugnot, C., Iliou, J.P., Privat, S., Robin, F., Vilaine, J.P. and Lenaers, A. (1992) J. Cardiovasc. Pharmacol. **20**, 340–347
106. Breugnot, C., Maziere, C., Auclair, M., Mora, L., Ronveaux, M.F., Salmon, S., Santus, R., Morliere, P., Lenaers, A. and Maziere, J.C. (1991) Free Radical Res. Commun. **15**, 91–100
107. Aviram, M., Dankner, G., Cogan, U., Hochgraf, E. and Brook, J.G. (1992) Metabolism **41**, 229–235
108. Giroux, L.M., Davignon, J. and Naruszewicz, M. (1993) Biochim. Biophys. Acta. **1165**, 335–338
109. Picard, S., Parthasarathy, S., Fruebis, J. and Witztum, J.L. (1992) Proc. Natl. Acad. Sci. U.S.A. **89**, 6876–6880
110. Fisher, M., Levine, P.H., Doyle, E.M., Arpano, M.M. and Hoogasian, J.J. (1991) Atherosclerosis **90**, 197–202
111. Breugnot, C., Maziere, C., Salmon, S., Auclair, M., Santus, R., Morliere, P., Lenaers, A. and Maziere, J.C. (1990) Biochem. Pharmacol. **40**, 1975–1980
112. Maziere, C., Auclair, M. and Maziere, J.C. (1992) Biochim. Biophys. Acta. **1126**, 314–318
113. Navab, M., Hama, S.Y., Van, L.B., Drinkwater, D.C., Laks, H. and Fogelman, A.M. (1993) J. Clin. Invest. **91**, 1225–1230
114. Kalant, N. and McCormick, S. (1992) Biochim. Biophys. Acta. **1128**, 211–219
115. Mackness, M.I., Arrol, S. and Durrington, P.N. (1991) FEBS Lett. **286**, 152–154
116. Stanton, L.W., White, R.T., Bryant, C.M., Protter, A.A. and Endemann, G. (1992) J. Biol. Chem. **267**, 22446–22451
117. Rankin, S.M., Knowles, M.E. and Leake, D.S. (1988) in Hyperlipidaemia and Atherosclerosis, pp. 214–215, Academic Press, London
118. Sparrow, C.P., Parthasarathy, S. and Steinberg, D. (1989) J. Biol. Chem. **264**, 2599–2604
119. Zhang, H., Basra, H.J.K. and Steinbrecher, U.P. (1990) J. Lipid Res. **31**, 1361–1369
120. Lougheed, M., Zhang, H. and Steinbrecher, U.P. (1991) J. Biol. Chem. **266**, 14519–14525
121. Jessup, W., Mander, E.L. and Dean, R.T. (1992) Biochim. Biophys. Acta. **1126**, 167–177
122. Roma, P., Bernini, F., Fogliatto, R., Bertulli, S.M., Negri, S., Fumagalli, R. and Catapano, A.L. (1992) J. Lipid Res. **33**, 819–829
122a. Mander, E.L., Dean, R.T., Stanley, K.K. and Jessup, W. (1994) Biochim. Biophys. Acta **1212**, 80–92
123. Jialal, I. and Chait, A. (1989) J. Lipid Res. **30**, 1561–1568
124. Simpson, J.A., Narita, S., Geiseg, S., Gebicki, S., Gebicki, J.M. and Dean, R.T. (1992) Biochem. J. **282**, 621–624
124a. Hoppe, G., O'Neil, J. and Hoff, H.F. (1994) J. Clin. Invest. **94**, 1506–1512
125. Grant, A.J., Jessup, W. and Dean, R.T. (1992) Biochim. Biophys. Acta. **1134**, 203–209
125a. Kritharides, L., Jessup, W. and Dean, R.T. (1995) Arteriosclerosis Thrombosis **15**, 276–289
126. Ball, R.Y., Bindman, J.P., Carpenter, K.L.H. and Mitchinson, M.J. (1986) Atherosclerosis **60**, 173–181
126a. Mitchinson, M.J., Hothersall, D.C., Brooks, P.N. and DeBarbure, C.Y. (1985) J. Pathol. **145**, 177.
127. Quinn, M.T., Parthasarathy, S. and Steinberg, D. (1988) Proc. Natl. Acad. Sci. U.S.A. **85**, 2805–2809
128. Autio, I., Jaakkola, O., Solakivi, T. and Nikkari, T. (1990) FEBS Lett. **277**, 247–249
129. Murugesan, G., Chisolm, G.M. and Fox, P.L. (1993) J. Cell Biol. **120**, 1011–1019

130. Lehr, H.A., Becker, M., Marklund, S.L., Hubner, C., Arsfors, K.E., Kohlschutter, A. and Messmer, K. (1992) Arteriosclerosis Thrombosis **12**, 824–829
131. Frostegard, J., Nilsson, J., Haegerstrand, A., Hamsten, A., Wigzell, H. and Gidlund, M. (1990) Proc. Natl. Acad. Sci. U.S.A. **87**, 904–908
132. Yui, S., Sasaki, T., Miyazaki, A., Horiuchi, S. and Yamasaki, M. (1993) Arteriosclerosis Thrombosis **13**, 331–337
133. Rosenfeld, M.E. and Ross, R. (1990) Arteriosclerosis **10**, 680–687
134. Morel, D.W., Hessler, J.R. and Chisolm, G.M. (1983) J. Lipid Res. **24**, 1070–1076
135. Reid, V.C. and Mitchinson, M.J. (1993) Atherosclerosis **98**, 17–24
136. Darley-Usmar, V.M., Severn, A., O'Leary, V.J. and Rogers, M. (1991) Biochem. J. **278**, 429–434
137. Aviram, M. (1989) Thromb. Res. **53**, 561–567
138. Latron, Y., Chautan, M., Anfosso, F., Alessi, M.C., Nalbone, G., Lafont, H. and Juhan-Vague, I. (1991) Arteriosclerosis Thrombosis **11**, 1821–1829
139. Weis, J.R., Pitas, R.E., Wilson, B.D. and Rodgers, G.M. (1991)FASEB J. **5**, 2459–2465
140. Wilson, B.D., Pitas, R.E. and Rodgers, G.M. (1992) Semin. Thromb. Hemost. **18**, 11–17
141. Weisser, B., Locher, R., Mengden, T. and Vetter, W. (1992) Arteriosclerosis Thrombosis **12**, 231–236
142. Negre-Salvayre, A., Fitoussi, G., Reaud, V., Pieraggi, M.-T., Thiers, J.-C. and Salvayre, R. (1992) FEBS Lett. **299**, 60–65
143. Chautan, M., Latron, Y., Anfosso, F., Alessi, M.-C., Lafont, H., Juhan-Vague, I. and Nalbone, G. (1993) J. Lipid Res. **34**, 101–110
144. Hirata, K., Akita, H. and Yokoyama, M. (1991) FEBS Lett. **287**, 181–184
145. Resink, T.J., Tkachuk, V.A., Bernhardt, J. and Buhler, F.R. (1992) Arteriosclerosis Thrombosis **12**, 278–285
146. Yokode, M., Kita, T., Kikawa, Y., Ogorochi, T., Narumiya, S. and Kawai, C. (1988) J. Clin. Invest. **81**, 720–729
147. Arai, H., Nagano, Y., Narumiya, S. and Kita, T. (1992) J. Biochem. (Tokyo) **112**, 482–487
148. Ek, B. and Humble, L. (1991) Biochem. Pharmacol. **41**, 695–699
149. Borsum, T., Henriksen, T. and Reisvag, A. (1985) Atherosclerosis **58**, 81–96
150. Fox, P.L., Chisolm, G.M. and DiCorleto, P.E. (1987) J. Biol. Chem. **262**, 6046–6054
151. Malden, L.T., Chait, A., Raines, E.W. and Ross, R. (1991) J. Biol. Chem. **266**, 13901–13907
152. Zwijsen, R.M.L., Japenga, S.C., Heijen, A.M.P., Van den Bos, R.C. and Koeman, J.H. (1992) Biochim. Biophys. Res. Commun. **186**, 1410–1416
153. Ross, R., Masuda, J., Raines, E.W., Gown, A.M., Katsuda, S., Sasahara, M., Malden, L.T., Masuko, H. and Sato, H. (1990) Science **248**, 1009–1012
154. Hamilton, T.A., Ma, G. and Chisolm, G.M. (1990) J. Immunol. **144**, 2343–2350
155. Ku, G., Thomas, C.E., Akeson, A.L. and Jackson, R.L. (1992) J. Biol. Chem. **267**, 14183–14188
156. Palinksi, W., Rosenfeld, M.E., Yla-Herttuala, S., Gurtner, G.C., Socher, S.S., Butler, S.W., Parthasarathy, S., Carew, T.E., Steinberg, D. and Witztum, J.L. (1989) Proc. Natl. Acad. Sci. U.S.A. **86**, 1372–1376
157. Parums, D.V., Brown, D.L. and Mitchinson, M.J. (1990) Arch. Pathol. Lab. Med. **114**, 383–387
158. Cushing, S.D., Berliner, J.A., Valente, A.J., Territo, M.C., Navab, M., Parhami, F., Gerrity, R., Schwartz, C.J. and Fogelman, A.M. (1990) Proc. Natl. Acad. Sci. U.S.A. **87**, 5134–5138
159. Drake, T.A., Hannani, K., Fei, H., Lavi, S. and Berliner, J.A. (1991) Am. J. Pathol. **138**, 601–607
160. Rajavashisth, T.B., Andalibi, A., Territo, M.C., Berliner, J.A., Navab, M., Fogelman, A.M. and Lusis, A.J. (1990) Nature **344**, 254–257
161. Chin, J.H., Azhar, S. and Hoffman, B.B. (1992) J. Clin. Invest. **89**, 10–18
162. Jorens, P.G., Rosseneu, M., Devreese, A.M., Bult, H., Marescau, B. and Herman, A.G. (1992) Eur. J. Pharmacol. **212**, 113–115
163. Wiklund, O., Mattsson, L., Bjornheden, T., Camejo, G. and Bondjers, G. (1991) J. Lipid Res. **32**, 55–62
164. Salonen, J.T., Salonen, R., Seppanen, K., Kartola, M., Suntioinen, S. and Korpela, H. (1991) Br. Med. J. **302**, 756–760

165. Salonen, J.T., Nyyssonen, K., Korpela, H., Tuomilehto, J., Seppanen, R. and Salonen, R. (1992) Circulation **86**, 808–811
166. Hunter, G.C., Dubick, M.A., Keen, C.L. and Eskelson, C.D. (1991) Proc. Soc. Exp. Biol. Med. **196**, 273–279
167. Smith, C., Mitchinson, M.J., Aruoma, O.I. and Halliwell, B. (1992) Biochem. J. **286**, 901–905
168. Balla, G., Jacob, H.S., Eaton, J.W., Belcher, J.D. and Vercellotti, G.M. (1991) Arteriosclerosis Thrombosis **11**, 1700–1711
169. Paganga, G., Rice-Evans, C., Rule, R. and Leake, D.S. (1992) FEBS Lett. **303**, 154–158
170. Lamb, D.J. and Leake, D.S. (1994) FEBS Lett. **352**, 15–18
171. Lamb, D.J. and Leake, D.S. (1994) FEBS Lett. **338**, 122–126
172. Smith, E.B. and Cochran, S. (1990) Atherosclerosis **84**, 173–181
173. Hurt-Camejo, E., Camejo, G., Rosengren, B., Lopez, F., Ahlstrom, C., Fager, G. and Bondjers, G. (1992) Arteriosclerosis Thrombosis **12**, 569–583
174. Navab, M., Imes, S.S., Hama, S.Y., Hough, G.P., Ross, L.A., Bork, R.W., Valente, A.J., Berliner, J.A., Drinkwater, D.C., Laks, H., et al. (1991) J. Clin. Invest. **88**, 2039–2046
175. Leake, D.S. (1991) Curr. Opin. Lipidol. **2**, 301–305

6

Ceroid, macrophages and atherosclerosis

M.J. Mitchinson*, K.L.H. Carpenter, J.V. Hunt, C.E. Marchant and V.C. Reid

Division of Cellular Pathology, University of Cambridge, Department of Pathology, Cambridge CB2 1QP, U.K.

Introduction

The best-known function of macrophages is scavenging, which involves both non-specific endocytosis and, even in invertebrates, receptor recognition of foreign material by lectin–sugar interactions. These mechanisms are conserved in mammals; but mammalian macrophages have evolved other functions whose sophistication is impressive and underestimated. It is often claimed that only the immune system can distinguish self from non-self; but macrophages can also do so. They will phagocytose foreign, senile or damaged cells but not healthy cells. Goldstein and Brown taught us that macrophages can preferentially endocytose abnormal large molecules, rather than their normal counterparts, and that one receptor, or group of receptors, can recognize molecules that have been altered in any of a variety of ways. This economical mechanism confers a versatility that presumably enables the survival even of animals without an immune system.

In addition, mammalian macrophages break down large foreign or waste molecules for recycling and for antigen presentation. They can also secrete a bewildering array of cytokines that affect the behaviour of nearby cells, such as in orchestrating wound healing. Their adaptability enables them to function in widely differing environments, such as in the high oxygen tension of alveoli and the near-anaerobic conditions of the edges of necrotic tissues. Their production of microbicidal oxygen radicals and catabolic enzymes has obvious protective effects which on occasion, however, when they spill into the tissues as in the pneumoconioses, can do more harm than good.

For all these reasons, the relatively recent realization that the foam cells of human atherosclerosis are macrophages has opened an era of atherosclerosis research which is as exciting as it is complicated.

---

* To whom correspondence should be addressed.

Ceroid in atherosclerosis

The insoluble lipid pigment, ceroid, was noticed in atherosclerotic plaques many years ago [1,2]. Ceroid occurs in tissues in a variety of circumstances, especially in vitamin E deficiency and, although varying in composition, always seems to be the result of oxidation of lipid–protein mixtures [3]. Ceroid is found in the necrotic base of advanced plaques, mainly in the form of rings or 'skins' around soluble lipid droplets, and, in early lesions, as granules and rings exclusively within the lipid-laden foam cells [4–6]. This prompted a hypothesis that foam cells were macrophages, that their microbicidal oxidative mechanisms led to lipoprotein oxidation, and that the result was the appearance not only of ceroid but perhaps also of diffusible lipid oxidation products with effects on plaque progression, including cytotoxicity [7].

Uptake of modified low-density lipoprotein by macrophages

At around the same time there was widespread interest in the recent discovery by Goldstein *et al.* that low-density lipoprotein (LDL) was taken up by macrophages, not via the LDL receptor, but mainly via a 'scavenger' pathway recognizing chemically altered proteins, including modified LDL [8]. This also supported the idea that foam cells were macrophages, since the scavenger pathway is not down-regulated, permitting the uptake of modified LDL in the large quantities necessary to create foam cells. Most forms of LDL modification producing this enhanced uptake seemed unlikely to occur *in vivo*, but one that quickly emerged as a likely candidate was oxidation.

It was initially shown that endothelial cells were capable of modifying LDL *in vitro* to enhance macrophage uptake [9]. There soon followed the discovery that not only endothelial cells [10,11], but also macrophages [12] and perhaps smooth muscle cells [13] were capable of contributing to LDL oxidation *in vitro*. Oxidation remains the most plausible explanation of LDL modification to enable foam cell formation *in vivo*, as referred to in other chapters; however, if it does occur, the exact sites and mechanisms of its formation remain uncertain.

It is also important to add that oxidation may not be the only form of LDL modification to occur *in vivo*; others, such as aggregation, or association with proteoglycans [14] may participate. Also, modified LDL may not be the only source of lipid accumulation in foam cells, although it is probably the main one.

Identification of human foam cells as macrophages

From Anitschkow onwards [15], there had always been a minority who favoured the idea that foam cells were macrophages. Ultrastructural and immunohistochemical studies have now demonstrated this beyond reasonable doubt [16–18]. Smooth muscle cells in the near vicinity, including the media, often also contain lipid droplets but, to judge from immunohistochemistry, never become so swollen as to lose their typical elongated shape. Therefore, if the term foam cells is reserved for cells so bloated with lipid as to be difficult to identify in conventional sections, all foam cells are macrophages.

Oxidized lipids and lipoproteins in human lesions

There are many reports of oxidation products of cholesterol and of other lipids in human atherosclerosis [19–21]. Most consistent has been the finding of cholest-5-en-3β,26-diol (or 26-hydroxycholesterol) and cholest-5-en-3β,7β-diol (or 7β-hydroxycholesterol), both recently found in gruel from advanced plaques, but not in normal arterial wall [22], and also found in earlier lesions, including fatty streaks (K.L.H. Carpenter, S.E. Taylor and M.J. Mitchinson, unpublished work).

Antibodies raised against various forms of oxidized LDL (oLDL) react with components of human lesions [23], suggesting that oLDL is present in atherosclerotic plaques, although possible cross-reactions with other forms of modified LDL remain a slight flaw in this argument [24].

Similarities between ceroid and oLDL

Artificial oxidation of LDL *in vitro* leads to the formation of floccules which, like ceroid, are insoluble, stain with lipid stains such as Oil Red O, show similar autofluorescence and have a similar multilamellar ultrastructure [6]. Both oLDL and ceroid are depleted in the oxidizable fatty acids: linoleate and arachidonate [6].

In many patients with advanced atherosclerosis, serum auto-antibodies reacting with ceroid are found; these cross-react with artificially oxidized LDL [25]. Finally, various antibodies to oLDL, when applied to histological sections or isolated foam cells, reveal ring-like structures in foam cells that bear a superficial resemblance to ceroid rings in human lesions [26].

These findings suggest the possibility that the ceroid found in human atherosclerosis may be composed at least partly of oLDL.

Depletion of linoleate and arachidonate

The depletion of linoleate (18:2) and arachidonate (20:4) but not oleate (18:1) in oLDL suggests they are being preferentially oxidized [6]. LDL extracted from human aorta has been shown to be depleted in linoleate [27]. Foam-cell-rich arterial lesions have smaller proportions of cholesteryl linoleate and arachidonate than either plasma LDL or fibrous lesions [28], suggesting that these two esters may be preferentially oxidized in the arterial wall, perhaps especially in foam cell-rich areas.

Oxidation of cholesteryl linoleate and arachidonate by macrophages *in vitro*

As mentioned before and more fully in other chapters, it has now been shown that LDL oxidation is enhanced by macrophages *in vitro*. However, human LDL is a complex particle, whose composition depends on a variety of factors, including the dietary content of various lipids and antioxidants. In an attempt to begin to dissect the process of LDL oxidation, we have therefore experimented with macrophages exposed to emulsions of a carrier protein (bovine serum albumin) with a single lipid species.

These experiments initially used only ceroid accumulation by the cells as a crude measure of oxidation of the emulsions. This showed the following. (i) All the emulsions tested, whatever the lipid used, were taken up rapidly by mouse peritoneal macrophages (MPM), which came to resemble foam cells. Scanning electron microscopy suggests that some of the particles of these artificial lipoproteins sink to the bottom of the dish and that the macrophages endocytose all they can reach (Fig. 1). (ii) There was no ceroid produced when the macrophages were cultured with emulsions containing cholesterol alone, or cholesteryl oleate or triolein [30]. (iii) Abundant ceroid granules accumulated when the cells were incubated with cholesteryl arachidonate [30]. (iv) Ceroid rings, or skins, around soluble lipid droplets were formed when the cells were cultured with cholesteryl linoleate [30]. These rings, and the granules mentioned above, were remarkably similar to those seen in human foam cells [6]. (v) Incubation with trilinolein or dilinolein also produced ceroid, but in coarse lumps quite unlike foam cells *in vivo* [30]. (vi) Pre-oxidation of cholesteryl linoleate before incubation with cells accelerated ceroid formation [30]. (vii) The radical-scavenging antioxidants, butylated hydroxytoluene, butylated hydroxyanisole [30] and probucol [31], virtually abolished ceroid formation from cholesteryl lineolate. (viii) The ultrastructure of ceroid formed in the MPM was similar to that seen in human foam cells [6,32]. (ix) A variety of different polyamino acid carriers, used instead of albumin, made little or no difference to the outcome [33]. (x) Human monocyte-

Fig. 1   **MPM in culture with medium containing cholesteryl arachidonate–bovine serum albumin emulsion, at 24 h**

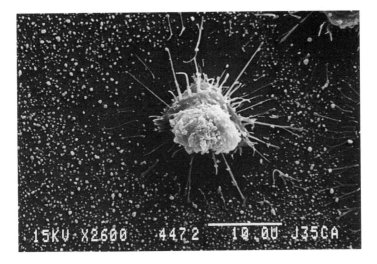

Scanning electron micrograph ×2600.

derived macrophages also produced ceroid from cholesteryl linoleate, but in smaller amounts than MPM [34].

These findings supported the idea that macrophages are capable of contributing to the oxidation of unsaturated lipids with at least two double bonds in the fatty acid side-chain (at least one bis-allylic carbon atom) and that the oxidation is at least partly due to free radicals. The results do not indicate, however, how much of the oxidation occurs before, and how much after, cell uptake.

Ceroid accumulation in macrophages, assessed by cytology, as evidence of cell-mediated oxidation of lipid–protein emulsions, has the merit that it reproduces an event which certainly occurs (although probably over a much longer time-scale) in atherosclerotic plaques, but it is only a crude method, unsuitable for quantitative assessment. This defect has been overcome by measuring the autofluorescence of ceroid in cell populations by flow cytometry [31,35]. This is proving to be a quick and convenient quantitative method to monitor the effects of changes in culture conditions and of various antioxidants upon cell-mediated oxidation of lipoproteins [35].

Lipid oxidation products in macrophage cultures

The accumulation of ceroid in mouse and human macrophages cultured with cholesteryl linoleate or cholesteryl arachidonate is accompanied by the appearance in the medium of 7β-hydroxycholesterol and hydroxyoctadecadienoic or hydroxyeicosatetraenoic acids, respectively [34,36], although the latter are in small and variable amounts, perhaps because of further catabolism. 7β-Hydroxycholesterol is consistently the most abundant oxidized lipid found in incubations with cholesteryl linoleate or cholesteryl arachidonate, but never with cholesteryl oleate or cholesterol alone.

This is of interest in suggesting a possible source for the 7β-hydroxycholesterol found in atherosclerotic plaques [20,22]. However, 26-hydroxycholesterol, which is even more abundant in the arterial lesions [22], has not been found in macrophage cultures. This may be because it results not from free radical activity, but from the action of cholesterol 26-hydroxylase, one of the enzymes of the P-450 group, which are said to be inactive in cultured cells [37].

The production of 7β-hydroxycholesterol by human macrophages is inhibited by probucol, α-tocopherol (vitamin E) and the metal chelator, EDTA [34] and is probably, at least in part, the result of metal ion-catalysed free radical activity. Copper and iron ions sufficient to fulfil this function are present *in vivo*, at least in advanced human lesions [38].

Cytotoxicity of macrophage-mediated lipoprotein oxidation

It has been known for some years that oxidation of LDL leads to cytotoxicity for a variety of cell types in culture, including endothelial cells, smooth muscle cells and fibroblasts [39]. This seems to be true both of LDL which has been oxidized artificially, such as by incubating with cupric sulphate, and also of LDL oxidized by cultured cells, including macrophages. The mechanisms of this toxicity and the molecules responsible have been little investigated, but there is clear evidence that certain oxysterols, including 7β-hydroxycholesterol, are cytotoxic *in vitro* [39], so the oxidation products of cholesterol are obvious candidates.

It has been speculated that such damage due to oLDL might be significant *in vivo*, especially because of the dangers of endothelial cell damage, including thrombosis [39]. However, it has not yet been detected *in vivo* whether such damage does occur in the lesion.

The 'missing link' in atherogenesis [40] is the onset of necrosis that eventually gives rise to the gruel, or atheroma, of the advanced lesion. How this comes about is hotly disputed, but to judge from immunohistochemistry, the cells dying to give rise to this mass are macrophage foam cells [17]. Occasional apparently dead or dying macrophages can be seen in the lower parts of collections of foam cells in small lesions; and, in most advanced lesions, the peripheral zone of foam cells at the 'shoulders' of the plaque shows dissolution of deeper cells, with spillage of antigen (and ceroid) into the necrotic base. Even before the immunohistochemical evidence, Schaefer had no doubt the necrotic zone was a 'graveyard of dead macrophages' [41].

It is therefore perhaps surprising that toxicity for macrophages has been little studied until recently. It was mentioned in one early report that macrophages were also vulnerable to oxysterols [42], but this was not investigated further.

LDL oxidized by cupric sulphate has now been shown to cause damage to mouse peritoneal macrophages that is evident almost immediately, assessed by tritiated adenine release *in vitro* [43]. Preincubation of the cells with physiologically relevant concentrations of α-tocopherol only delayed this toxicity slightly [43]. Perhaps more importantly, native LDL caused similar toxicity, but only after a delay of 20 h [43]. Preincubation of the cells with α-tocopherol reduced this damage significantly, the findings suggesting that oxidation of LDL by the macrophages themselves was producing this toxicity [43]. By 24 h, the damage caused by native LDL was as severe as that caused by oLDL [43].

Similar toxicity is seen when MPM are incubated with emulsions containing cholesteryl linoleate or cholesteryl arachidonate, but not with cholesteryl oleate [44]. Knowing from previous work that this tallies with the capacity of MPM to oxidize these particles [30], it was no surprise to find that α-tocopherol, incorporated into the emulsions, also protected against this toxicity [44].

Thus there is evidence *in vitro* that the process of macrophage-mediated LDL oxidation is toxic for the macrophages themselves, and that this self-inflicted toxicity might be due to oxidation of certain cholesteryl esters in the LDL particle. Obviously other, so far untested, components of LDL might also be involved. However, recent experiments have shown that 7β-hydroxycholesterol is toxic for macrophages (V.C. Reid and M.J. Mitchinson, unpublished work), and the oxidation products of cholesterol remain likely culprits.

Morphology of macrophage toxicity

The toxicity of oLDL, or oxidizable cholesteryl esters *in vitro*, is obvious even by light microscopy, but electron microscopy produced a total surprise. Scanning electron microscopy showed loss of surface ruffles, as well as blebbing and pitting of the plasma membrane, all of which were not unexpected. However, transmission electron microscopy of the damaged cultures showed numerous cells with characteristic changes not of necrosis, but of apoptosis. These include condensation of nuclear chromatin into peripheral densities, nucleolar dissolution, swelling of the rough endoplasmic reticulum, condensation and characteristic outbuddings of the viable-looking cytoplasm, with preservation of organelles, including mitochondria [45]. The remaining characteristic of apoptosis — which is DNA cleavage, or 'laddering', dependent on endonuclease activity — is also demonstrable [46].

Apoptosis was originally described as the changes, distinct from necrosis, that are found in 'programmed cell death' occurring in tissues during the remodellings of ontogeny, including the immune system, in the regular cell turnover of tissues such as gut epithelium, and in neoplasms [47]. An important feature of apoptosis, in addition to the morphological and DNA changes mentioned above, is that it requires synthesis of cell proteins, including nucleases. It is therefore an active process, cell suicide, rather than a passive injury. However, a number of examples have now emerged of apoptosis that is not 'programmed', but caused by exogenous chemicals: one example is the death of lymphocytes *in vitro* due to oxysterols [48]. The similarity to the recent findings in macrophages is obvious, but the explanation of the phenomenon is lacking.

Foam cell apoptosis has not been described in previous ultrastructural studies of atherosclerosis, but it may be wise to look again.

Significance of macrophage toxicity

If the events described above occur *in vivo*, this could be of importance. The presence of basal necrosis is a dominant feature of advanced atherosclerosis and is certainly unusual in human pathology because it appears not to elicit the usual inflammatory response and healing. There are those who believe that the onset of necrosis marks the onset of irreversibility [49]. This may be an exaggerated claim but it is at least, in all probability, an important step in conferring bulk and friability to the lesions, and enhancing the risk of thrombosis.

In addition, catabolic enzymes spilled from dead macrophages may well contribute to secondary medial damage. This can result in atherosclerotic aneurysm formation, as well as the auto-allergic inflammation known as chronic periaortitis [50], which is accompanied by auto-antibodies to ceroid, as mentioned above [25].

Macrophages, ceroid and α-tocopherol

Our own work has been confined to investigation of the hypothesis that macrophage foam cells contribute to the oxidation of components of LDL, with the production of ceroid and oxidized lipids, and resultant toxicity for the macrophages themselves. These three events *in vitro* do correspond with evidence gleaned from human atherosclerotic lesions, and all three are inhibited by α-tocopherol *in vitro*. This in turn suggests an explanation for at least part of the protective effects of dietary antioxidant supplements in experimental animals [51], including α-tocopherol in primates [52].

The main significance of ceroid *in vitro* is that it acts as an easily detectable marker for the end-stages of lipoprotein oxidation and therefore can be used as an alternative to the many other ways of assessing that oxidation. *In vivo* it is presumably chemically inert, but it is conceivable that it might hinder dispersion of lipid droplets, and it is antigenic [25]. However, macrophages may have many other functions in the development of atherosclerosis.

Other potential roles of macrophages

There is now an abundant literature on other macrophage functions *in vitro* that might play a part in atherogenesis. Some of the more attractive examples follow. (i) Macrophage-derived growth factor might cause smooth muscle cell replication and attract smooth muscle cells into the intima, in a way analogous to the role of macrophages in wound healing [53,54]. (ii) Macrophages might cause the change of phenotype of smooth muscle cells from contractile to secretory [55]. (iii) Macrophage chemotactic protein-1 might influence recruitment of more monocytes [56]. (iv) LDL oxidized by macrophages is a chemoattractant for monocytes, but arrests macrophage migration, thus potentially trapping macrophages in the lesion [57]. (v) Macrophage foam cells might leave the lesions by re-entering the blood. This has not been proved, but is an obvious possible explanation for regression [58]. (vi) Macrophages might present antigen to T-lymphocytes in the lesion and in turn be stimulated by lymphokines [59]. (vii) Cytokines secreted by macrophages might be capable of inducing adhesion molecules on endothelial cells [60]. (viii) Macrophages might stimulate ingrowth of vasa vasorum [61].

There is no shortage of data obtained *in vitro* on the effects of macrophage-derived molecules, such as cytokines and eicosanoids, on endothelial and smooth muscle cells. Which of them are significant *in vivo* is more difficult to establish.

Accelerated atherosclerosis in diabetes mellitus

The acceleration of atherosclerosis seen in diabetes has often been suspected to be related to the modification of LDL caused by glycation [62]. Recent findings raise the distinct possibility that the important modification might not simply be glycation, but oxidative sequelae engendered by glycation [62–65].

Overview of the role of macrophages in atherogenesis

The diffuse intimal thickening of advancing age is composed of secretory smooth muscle cells. This process is accentuated in a wide variety of conditions, including intimal 'cushions' at branching points and in reaction to such insults as hypertension, immune complex deposition, chronic rejection, irradiation and many others. This common reaction of the artery to injury does not involve macrophages, never undergoes necrosis, does not usually significantly narrow the lumen and does not usually precipitate thrombosis or major ischaemia.

What distinguishes the focal lesions of atherosclerosis is the presence of macrophages. Given the present state of knowledge, it seems that their activity leads to progression of the lesions. This suggests that atherosclerosis is a chronic inflammatory disease in which (as in the pneumoconioses) the macrophage is doing more harm than good. The role of smooth muscle cells, as in the conditions mentioned above, may be purely reparative, like fibroblasts in a healing wound.

The site of oxidation of LDL *in vivo* is still not certain. It could be seeded by oxidized lipids in the diet, or some oxidation might occur in the blood. The evidence at present, however, suggests it mainly occurs in the artery wall. Whether this oxidation in the wall is cell-mediated, and whether it is extracellular or intracellular is not known; however, it is certainly possible that oxidation begins at the surface of a macrophage due to its surface production of free radicals, and that this enhances uptake and subsequent further oxidation within the macrophage. One of the findings that favours this scenario is that ceroid and oxidized lipids (including 7β-hydroxy- and 26-hydroxycholesterol) are also present in pulmonary artery atherosclerosis (S.E. Taylor, K.L.H. Carpenter and M.J. Mitchinson, unpublished work). Extracellular oxidation seems less likely in the lower oxygen tensions of the pulmonary artery and, as mentioned earlier, macrophages are apparently capable of deploying their oxidative activity even in low oxygen environments.

Implications for the population

Epidemiological evidence for a protective effect of dietary antioxidants and antioxidant supplements has been described. The clear implication is that many industrialized populations have a diet deficient in antioxidants. Various trials of the effect of antioxidant supplements on subsequent complications of atherosclerosis are now proceeding. It is not difficult, however, to detect nervousness in some quarters about the implications of what might emerge. Is it conceivable that the populations at risk could be advised to take prophylactic dietary supplements? At first sight, there appears to be no precedent, but alien human environments have often demanded such measures. No one questioned the advisability of taking fruits on long sea journeys or providing astronauts with oxygen. If we wish to continue to live in the alien environment of industrialized societies, and not suffer the complications of atherosclerosis, similar precautions would be justifiable, in our view. The evidence required to establish that justification clearly, however, is not yet available.

We are grateful for the collaboration and advice of Dr J. Skepper, J. Skamarauskas and other colleagues; and for the assistance of V. Mullins.

References

1. Pappenheimer, A.M. and Victor, J. (1946) Am. J. Pathol. **22**, 395–413
2. Burt, R.C. (1952) Am. J. Clin. Pathol. **22**, 135–139
3. Wolman, M. (1975) Isr. J. Med. Sci. **11** (Suppl.)
4. Mitchinson, M.J. (1982) Atherosclerosis **45**, 11–15
5. Mitchinson, M.J., Hothersall, D.C., Brooks, P.N. and de Burbure, C.Y. (1985) J. Pathol. **145**, 177–183
6. Ball, R.Y., Carpenter, K.L.H. and Mitchinson, M.J. (1987) Arch. Pathol. **111**, 1134–1140
7. Mitchinson, M.J. (1983) Med. Hypotheses **12**, 171–178
8. Goldstein, J.L., Ho, Y.K., Basu, S.K. and Brown, M.S. (1979) Proc. Natl. Acad. Sci. U.S.A. **76**, 333–337
9. Henriksen, T., Mahoney, E.M. and Steinberg, D. (1981) Proc. Natl. Acad. Sci. U.S.A. **78**, 6499–6503
10. Morel, D.W., DiCorleto, P.E. and Chisolm, G.M. (1984) Arteriosclerosis **4**, 357–364
11. Steinbrecher, U.P., Parthasarathy, S., Leake, D.S., Witztum, J.L. and Steinberg, D. (1984) Proc. Natl. Acad. Sci. U.S.A. **81**, 3883–3887
12. Cathcart, M.K., Morel, D.W. and Chisolm, G.M. (1985) J. Leukocyte Biol. **38**, 341–350
13. Heinecke, J.W., Rosen, H. and Chait, A. (1984) J. Clin. Invest. **74**, 1890–1894
14. Vijayagopal, P., Srinivasan, S.R., Radhakrishnamurthy, B. and Berenson, G.S. (1993) Biochem. J. **289**, 837–844
15. Anitschkow, N. (1933) in Arteriosclerosis: A Survey of the Problem (Cowdry, E.V., ed.), pp. 271–322, Macmillan, New York
16. Gerrity, R.G. (1981) Am. J. Path. **103**, 181–190
17. Aqel, N., Ball, R.Y., Waldmann, H. and Mitchinson, M.J. (1985) J. Pathol. **146**, 197–204
18. Stary, H.C. (1989) Arteriosclerosis **9** (Suppl. 1), 19–32
19. Glavind, J., Hartmann, S., Clemmesen, J., Jessen, K.E. and Dam, H. (1952) Acta. Pathol. Microbiol. Scand. **30**, 1–6
20. Brooks, C.J.W., Steel, G., Gilbert, J.D. and Harland, W.A. (1971) Atherosclerosis **13**, 223–237
21. Harland, W.A., Gilbert, J.D. and Brooks, C.J.W. (1973) Biochim. Biophys. Acta **316**, 378–385
22. Carpenter, K.L.H., Taylor, S.E., Ballantine, J.A., Fussell, B., Halliwell, B. and Mitchinson, M.J. (1993) Biochim. Biophys. Acta. **1167**, 121–130
23. Ylä-Herttuala, S., Palinski, W., Rosenfeld, M.E., Parthasarathy, S., Carew, T.E., Butler, S., Witztum, J.L. and Steinberg, D. (1989) J. Clin. Invest. **84**, 1086–1095
24. Leading Article (1992) Lancet **339**, 899–900
25. Parums, D.V., Brown, D.L. and Mitchinson, M.J. (1990) Arch. Pathol. **114**, 383–387
26. Rosenfeld, M.E., Khoo, J.C., Miller, E., Parthasarathy, S., Palinski, W. and Witztum, J.L (1991) J. Clin. Invest. **87**, 90–99
27. Hoff, H.F. and Gaubatz, J.W. (1982) Atherosclerosis **42**, 273–279
28. Smith, E.B., Evans, P.H. and Downham, M.D. (1967) J. Atheroscler. Res. **7**, 171–186

29. Ball, R.Y., Bindman, J.P., Carpenter, K.L.H. and Mitchinson, M.J. (1986) Atherosclerosis 60, 173–181
30. Ball, R.Y., Carpenter, K.L.H., Enright, J.H., Hartley, S.L. and Mitchinson, M.J. (1987) Br. J. Exp. Pathol. 68, 427–438
31. Carpenter, K.L.H., Ball, R.Y., Carter, N.P., Woods, S.E., Hartley, S.L., Davies, S., Enright, J.H. and Mitchinson, M.J. (1990) Adv. Exp. Med. Biol. 266, 333–343
32. Ball, R.Y., Carpenter, K.L.H. and Mitchinson, M.J. (1988) Br. J. Exp. Pathol. 69, 43–56
33. Ardeshna, K.M., Ball, R.Y., Carpenter, K.L.H., Enright, J.H. and Mitchinson, M.J. (1990) Int. J. Exp. Pathol. 71, 799–808
34. Carpenter, K.L.H., Ballantine, J.A., Fussell, B., Enright, J.H. and Mitchinson, M.J. (1990) Atherosclerosis 83, 217–229
35. Hunt, J.V., Carpenter, K.L.H., Bottoms, M.A., Carter, N.P., Marchant, C.E. and Mitchinson, M.J. (1993) Atherosclerosis 98, 229–239
36. Carpenter, K.L.H., Ball, R.Y., Ardeshna, K.M., Bindman, J.P., Enright, J.H., Hartley, S.L., Nicholson, S. and Mitchinson, M.J. (1988) in Lipofuscin 1987: State of the Art (Nagy, I.Z., ed.), pp. 245–268, Elsevier, Amsterdam
37. Benford, D.J. and Hubbard, S.A. (1987) in Biochemical Toxicology: A Practical Approach (Snell, K. and Mullock, B., eds.), pp. 68–69, I.R.L. Press, Oxford
38. Smith, C., Mitchinson, M.J., Aruoma, O.I. and Halliwell, B. (1992) Biochem. J. 286, 901–905
39. Chisolm, G.M. (1991) Curr. Opin. Lipidol. 2, 311–316
40. McGill, H.C., Jr. (1990) in Pathobiology of the Human Atherosclerotic Plaque (Glagov, S., Newman, W.P. III and Schaffer, S.A., eds.), pp. 1–11, Springer-Verlag, New York
41. Schaefer, H.-E. (1981) in Disorders of the Monocyte–Macrophage System (Schmaltzl, F., Huhn, D. and Schaefer, H.-E., eds.), pp. 137–142, Springer–Verlag, Berlin
42. Baranowski, A., Adams, C.W.M., Bayliss High, O.B. and Bowyer, D.E. (1982) Atherosclerosis 41, 255–266
43. Reid, V.C. and Mitchinson, M.J. (1993) Atherosclerosis 98, 17–24
44. Reid, V.C., Brabbs, C.E. and Mitchinson, M.J. (1992) Atherosclerosis 92, 251–260
45. Reid, V.C., Mitchinson, M.J. and Skepper, J.N. (1993) J. Pathol. 171, 321–328
46. Reid, V.C., Hardwick, S.J and Mitchinson, M.J. (1993) FEBS Letts. 332, 218–220
47. Carson, D.A. and Ribeiro, J.M. (1993) Lancet 341, 1251–1254
48. Christ, M., Luu, B., Mejia, J.E., Moosbrugger, I. and Bischoff, P. (1993) Immunology 78, 455–460
49. Velican, C. and Velican, D. (1981) Atherosclerosis 39, 479–496
50. Mitchinson, M.J. (1986) Arch. Pathol. 110, 784–786
51. Jialal, I. and Scaccini, C. (1992) Curr. Opin. Lipidol. 3, 324–328
52. Verlangieri, A. and Bush, M. (1992) J. Am. Coll. Nutr. 11, 131–138
53. Martinet, Y., Bitterman, P.B., Mornex, J.-F., Grotendorst, G.R., Martin, G.R. and Crystal, R.G. (1986) Nature (London) 319, 158–160
54. Nilsson, J. (1986) Atherosclerosis 62, 185–199
55. Rennick, R.E., Campbell, J.H. and Campbell, G.R. (1988) Atherosclerosis 71, 35–43
56. Ylä-Herttuala, S., Lipton, B.A., Rosenfeld, M.E., Särkioja, T., Yoshimura, T., Leonard, E.J., Witztum, J.L. and Steinberg, D. (1991) Proc. Natl. Acad. Sci. U.S.A. 88, 5252–5256
57. Quinn, M.T., Parthasarathy, S., Fong, L.G. and Steinberg, D. (1987) Proc. Natl. Acad. Sci. U.S.A. 84, 2995–2998
58. Gerrity, R.G. (1981) Am. J. Pathol. 103, 191–200
59. Libby, P. and Hansson, G.K. (1991) Lab. Invest. 64, 5–15
60. Poston, R.N., Haskard, D.O., Coucher, J.R., Gall, N.P. and Johnson-Tidey, R.R. (1992) Am. J. Pathol. 140, 665–673
61. Polverini, P.J., Cotran, R.S. Gimbrone, M.A., Jr. and Unanue, E.R. (1977) Nature (London) 269, 804–806
62. Lyons, T.J. (1992) Diabetes 41 (Suppl. 2), 67–73
63. Hunt, J.V., Dean, R.T. and Wolff, S.P. (1988) Biochem. J. 256, 205–212
64. Hunt, J.V., Smith, C.C.T. and Wolff, S.P. (1990) Diabetes 39, 1420–1424
65. Hunt, J.V., Bottoms, M.A. and Mitchinson, M.J. (1993) Biochem. J. 291, 529–535

7

Vascular responses during the development of athero-sclerosis and lipoprotein oxidation

Michael Jacobs* and K. Richard Bruckdorfer†

Departments of *Pharmacology and †Biochemistry, Royal Free Hospital
School of Medicine, Rowland Hill Street, London NW3 2PF, U.K.

Introduction

The normal functions of the heart and blood vessels depend critically on the regulatory mechanisms that maintain blood pressure and prevent blood clotting. In recent years, it has become apparent that the inner layer of cells that lines the blood vessel wall, namely the endothelium, plays a pivotal role by secreting regulators of blood coagulation and blood flow. It is therefore not surprising that atherosclerosis, a complex disease of the vessel wall which is thought to involve lipoproteins and platelets, modifies these regulatory processes. This chapter describes how the regulation of constriction and dilatation of the artery wall are influenced by the development of atherosclerosis and emphasizes the role of oxidation of lipoproteins and the aggregation of platelets.

One of the most important regulators of blood pressure and platelet aggregation, endothelium-derived relaxing factor, turns out to be the very simple molecule, nitric oxide (NO). NO is a very pervasive molecule with ubiquitous functions which have been extensively reviewed [1,2]. Another mediator released from the endothelium with similar functions is a product of the cyclo-oxygenase pathway, prostacyclin (PGI_2) [2]. At a local level, these substances contribute to the regulation of vascular tone, countering angiotensin II and endothelin, the major vasoconstrictors released from the endothelium [2].

Mediators of endothelium-dependent vasodilatation and platelet aggregation

Endothelium-dependent vasodilatation depends predominantly on the release of NO [1,2] by flow-mediated activation of calcium-dependent potassium channels [3] and stimulation of endothelial receptors by endogenous vasodilators. Although flow-mediated release of PGI_2 from the endothelium has been demonstrated [4], it appears to be less important than NO in endothelium-dependent vasodilatation [5]. NO and PGI_2 are also implicated in haemostasis, where their role is to act synergistically to inhibit platelet adhesion and aggregation [1,2]. The patency of the collateral circulation, which is so vital in protecting the heart when ischaemia and infarction occur, is also maintained by the production of NO [6].

L-Arginine:NO pathway

NO is synthesized in endothelial cells from L-arginine by a calcium-dependent constitutive isoform of the enzyme nitric oxide synthase (cNOS) and stimulates the soluble guanylate cyclase of the vascular smooth muscle to induce relaxation (Fig. 1).

A calcium-independent isoform of NO synthase (iNOS) can be induced in a variety of cells [1], including macrophages, by cytokines [7]. The macrophage enzyme contains tightly bound calcium–calmodulin and is regulated by the availability of L-arginine [8]. This is in contrast to the constitutive endothelial isoform which is switched on by the elevation of cytosolic calcium. Normally, NOS is absent from vascular smooth muscle cells but is induced in diseases such as septic shock [9], whereas cNOS is upregulated in endothelial cells by shear stress [10]. Thus, the L-arginine: NO pathway in the cardiovascular system, under normal physiological conditions and in disease, will continuously utilize L-arginine.

PGI₂ biosynthesis

PGI_2 is the principal product of the cyclo-oxygenase pathway in the endothelium, although it is also synthesized in substantial amounts by other cells in the artery wall. It is biosynthesized from arachidonic acid, originating from membrane phospholipids, through the prostaglandin endoperoxides which are the substrates for PGI_2 synthase. Some prostaglandin endoperoxides may be obtained from activation of platelets. The principal effect of PGI_2 is through receptor-mediated processes, which bring about an inhibition of platelet aggregation and the relaxation of the smooth muscle through an increase in intracellular cyclic AMP [2]. This prostaglandin may, therefore, be of key importance in the prevention of thrombosis associated with the clinical presentation of cardiovascular disease.

Endothelium-dependent vasodilatation and atherosclerosis

Endothelium-dependent vasodilatation can be demonstrated in an organ bath by eliciting the relaxation of a preconstricted isolated arterial ring segment

Fig. 1   L-Arginine:NO pathway

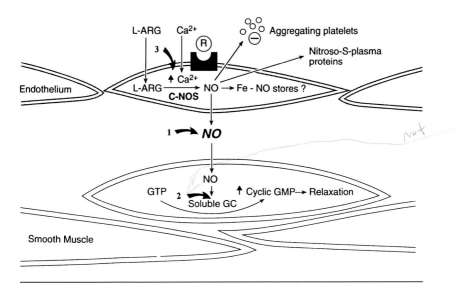

Possible sites of inhibition by oxidized lipoproteins are shown: (1) direct binding/inactivation of NO [55,58]; (2) inhibition of soluble guanylate cyclase [55,68,69]; (3) inhibition of production and release of NO [55,56,66]. Abbreviations used: L-ARG, L-arginine; GC, guanylate cyclase; C-NOS, constitutive NO synthase.

with agents that release NO from the endothelium, as was done with acetylcholine (ACh) in the classical experiments performed by Furchgott and Zawadzki [11]. When rings are obtained from isolated animal arteries with experimentally induced atherosclerosis, relaxations are invariably reduced. These latter observations are confirmed by studies showing that patients with coronary artery disease have impaired vasodilatation and often show a vasoconstriction to infusion of ACh into their coronary arteries [12]. These alterations in vascular reactivity will affect the protective responses to flow conditions and arterial occlusion and lead to damage of the vessel wall.

The purpose of this chapter is to compare the alterations in vascular reactivity in human coronary artery disease with those found in experimental models of developing atherosclerosis and to examine the role of lipoproteins, particularly oxidized low-density lipoprotein (oLDL) and platelets, in these dysfunctions.

Impaired vasodilatation in human coronary artery disease and experimental atherosclerosis

Clinical studies

Numerous angiographic studies [12] have demonstrated that the infusion of ACh into large atherosclerotic coronary arteries [13], and arteries that appear normal but have more diffuse atherosclerosis [14], causes a shift from the normal ACh-induced vasodilatation to a vasoconstriction. These dysfunctions appear to correlate with risk factors for coronary heart disease including age, hypertension, plasma cholesterol level [13,15,16] and LDL concentration [15]. Flow-induced increases in vasodilatation in these arteries are also reduced in atherosclerotic arteries [17,18], but are preserved in those from hypercholesterolaemic patients at the early stages of atherosclerosis [16]. Usually endothelium-independent vasodilatation to nitrovasodilators is unaffected by atherosclerosis, suggesting the defect is not due to inhibition of the soluble guanylate cyclase of the smooth muscle [12,13–15]. The action of papaverine, another endothelium-independent vasodilator is surprisingly inhibited [16]. A detailed study by Zeiher *et al.* [15] has suggested that a gradual impairment of vasodilatation to different stimuli occurs as coronary artery disease progresses, commencing at an early stage of the disease with the selective dysfunction of receptor-mediated, endothelium-dependent, relaxation and progressing to a complete loss of NO responses to all stimuli.

Animal models

The observations found in these clinical studies are largely confirmed in experimental models of atherosclerosis using isolated arteries of primates [19], pigs [20] and rabbits [21,22–25]. In some studies of isolated arteries from hypercholesterolaemic animals, endothelium-dependent relaxations evoked by ACh and 5-hydroxytryptamine (5-HT) are selectively impaired, whereas dilator responses to bradykinin, substance P and the calcium ionophore A23187 are preserved [22]. In contrast, Galle *et al.* [23] found that impairment was closely correlated with the degree of intimal thickening and was absent in hypercholesterolaemia alone. In severe atherosclerosis, inhibition of NO responses by all stimulants seems to occur.

Impairment in resistance vessels

Although the impairment of vasodilatation in large vessels may be important in vasospasm and highly stenosed arteries, it is unlikely to contribute to the regulation of blood flow in the heart which is determined by the resistance vessels. These microvessels exhibit impaired flow in patients, which correlates with hypercholesterolaemia or advanced age irrespective of epicardial atherosclerosis or hypertension [16]. Similar impairment of endothelium-dependent vasodilatation in the human forearm resistance vessels has also been demonstrated in hypercholesterolaemic patients [26]. Perfused rabbit heart [27] and hindlimb beds [28] show attenuated, endothelium-dependent relaxation mediated by the release of NO, as do isolated coronary resistance vessels [29,30]. Since the resistance vessels show only minor alterations in endothelial cell morphology [31], even if the large arteries have intimal thickening, it suggests that hypercholesterolaemia *per se* inhibits NO responses. Furthermore, the impairment of microvessels by hypercholesterolaemia also extends to collateral blood vessels whose formation is induced by arterial occlusion [32]

Mechanisms underlying the alteration in NO-dependent vasodilatation

The impairment of NO responses described above could occur at numerous steps between activation of the L-arginine:NO pathway via elevation of intracellular calcium and relaxation of the smooth muscle as shown in Fig. 1. The majority of studies *in vivo* point to a step before activation of guanylate cyclase, since most studies have found that endothelium-independent vasodilatation by nitrovasodilators is unaffected by hypercholesterolaemia [12] and all but the most severe atherosclerosis [33]. This view has been confirmed using a bioassay technique with a donor endothelialized artery stimulated with ACh to produce NO and a detector arterial ring, with or without endothelium, to measure the NO response [33]. By using different combinations of normal/atherosclerotic arteries, it was shown that NO was released normally and probably inactivated prior to its action on guanylate cyclase. This was confirmed in a study by Minor *et al.* [34] showing that release of NO from atherosclerotic aorta, as measured by chemiluminescence, was increased despite the fact that endothelium-dependent relaxations were reduced. In hypercholesterolaemia, A23187-evoked relaxations were unchanged in contrast to their reduction in atherosclerosis. Flavahan [22] has argued that the impairment of relaxation evoked by ACh and 5-HT, but not A23187, in hypercholesterolaemia is due to a defect in signal transduction involving desensitization of pertussis-sensitive G_i-protein. Alternatively, this may be explained by the large increase in NO produced (two-fold greater than from a normal artery [34]) by A23187 stimulation and/or a lower release of free radicals that inactivate NO. One can speculate that the increase in flow and stimulated release of NO (calcium-dependent processes) by hypercholesterolaemia and atherosclerosis results from an upregulation of the expression of cNOS, which is also known to be induced by shear stress [6]. iNOS may also be expressed, since L-arginine can reverse the impairment of NO responses in the human coronary arteries of hypercholesterolaemic patients [35], and in the perfused hindlimb [36] and isolated aorta [37] of hypercholesterolaemic rabbits. There is some support for this view from a study showing that calcium-independent

NOS, presumably iNOS, is present in the lung tissue of hypercholesterol-aemic rabbits [38]. Cultured smooth muscle cells enriched with cholesterol [39] from exposure to modified LDL, also show enhanced production of NO. It is, however, far from clear that normal or increased NO will be produced continually during the development of atherosclerosis. In fact, several studies have indicated that the impairment of relaxation in atherosclerotic aorta is not reversed by incubation with L-arginine [40] or by prior dietary supplementa-tion with the amino acid (P. Kerr and M. Jacobs, unpublished work), in con-trast to the findings of Cooke *et al.* [37]. Furthermore, it is possible that NO itself inhibits guanylate cyclase [41,42] or down-regulates iNOS [41] and oLDL prevents the expression of iNOS [43]. Investigations of the expression of NOS using cDNA probes and specific antibodies for NOS should clarify these studies in the near future.

What are the factors that inactivate NO in vessels that are exposed to hypercholesterolaemia or contain atherosclerotic lesions? Considerable evi-dence points to the inactivation of NO by superoxide anions [33,34], which are produced in greater amounts by the aorta of hypercholesterolaemic rabbits than by the aorta of normal rabbits [44]. Superoxide may be produced intra-cellularly, since polyethylene glycolated superoxide dismutase (a form of the enzyme which can enter cells or bind to the glycocalyx [45]) significantly improves endothelium-dependent relaxation. A further consequence of excess production of superoxide anions may be to increase lipid peroxidation of LDL and accelerate the atherosclerotic process. The interaction of lipopro-teins with NO may also have another dimension, in relation to the potential of NO to act as an antioxidant or pro-oxidant during the oxidation of these lipoproteins. These possibilities are discussed in detail in Chapter 4.

The influence of plasma lipoproteins on vasodilatation

General

Exposure of the arterial wall to LDL leads to a rapid accumulation of LDL-like particles and aggregates that are enmeshed in the extracellular matrix at focal areas prone to atherosclerotic lesions [46]. During the development of atherosclerosis, these lipoproteins become oxidized, leading to the formation of fatty streaks and more complex lesions. Thus, accumulation of LDL in the intima is a probable factor in the impairment of coronary vasodilatation. This agrees with the finding that the dysfunction is related to elevated plasma chol-esterol [13] and LDL concentrations [15] and is negatively correlated with plasma high-density lipoprotein (HDL) [47]. Furthermore, the cholesterol-lowering drug lovastatin will prevent impairment in the aorta [23] and in the isolated perfused heart from cholesterol-fed animals [48]. The antioxidants γ-tocopherol [49] and probucol [50] also suppress the impairment of NO responses, implicating the oxidative modification of LDL. It is therefore possible that exposure of isolated arteries to LDL in the organ bath might mimic the inhibition of NO responses occurring in hypercholesterolaremia, whereas exposure to oLDL might resemble more the situation in the atherosclerotic lesion, where there is continuous production of LDL peroxidation products. It should be realized, however, that lipoproteins — and human LDL in particular — are a heterogenous mixture of macromolecules that differ in composition between individuals. In addition, preparations of oLDL will also vary in composition according to the conditions of oxidation [51]. Therefore, studies of the effects of lipoproteins on cellular functions have many pitfalls [52] and require careful characterization of the native and oxidized lipoproteins to enable results to be compared.

LDL

Inhibition of NO-mediated, endothelium-dependent relaxation by native LDL has not been found consistently [53–62]. However, the inhibition can only be attributed to the native lipoproteins when there is evidence that significant oxidative modification is absent. If stringent precautions are taken during the preparation of LDL, only trace amounts of lipid peroxides are present [63], whereas micromolar concentrations are required to cause a small reversible inhibition of relaxation [64]. Interestingly, native LDL which had no detectable oxidation, was unable to inhibit the relaxations of rabbit aortic rings precontracted with phenylephrine [55]. However, if noradrenaline or 5-HT was used to precontract the tissues, a reversible inhibition was seen [55]. This suggests that, in the presence of these readily oxidizable agonists, peroxidation is promoted and sufficient lipid peroxides are produced to cause an inhibition. The role of oxidation was confirmed by the fact that antioxidants such as ascorbic acid and probucol were able to abolish the inhibition [57].

oLDL

Copper- and endothelial cell-induced oxidation of LDL inhibit endothelium-dependent relaxation in large arteries more potently than native LDL [54–61]. LDL oxidized by copper also inhibits NO responses in rabbit coronary resistance vessels [65]. There are some suggestions that the inhibition is selective for relaxations evoked by 5-HT in porcine coronary arteries [66] and responses evoked by A23187 are less affected [60,67], as occurs in hypercholesterolaemia.

Reports on the site of action of oLDL are contradictory and may reflect multiple sites of action (Fig. 1; [55,56,58,66,68,69]).

This complexity is not surprising, since different conditions have been used for the oxidation and these will critically determine the inhibitory constituents of the final oLDL. If preparations of oLDL from individual donors are used, considerable variation in inhibitory potency is found [56].

The oLDL preparations from the majority of donors inhibited relaxation reversibly, while a few donors inhibited more potently and irreversibly. The potency of the inhibition correlated positively with the susceptibility of the original LDL to oxidation by copper (Fig. 2) [56]. The susceptibility of LDL

Fig. 2   **Scattergram showing the relationship between the susceptibility to oxidation of LDL from different donors and inhibition of relaxation by their oLDL**

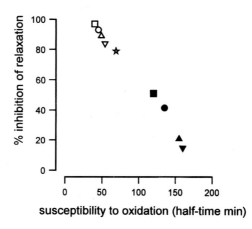

Data taken from [56].

to oxidation is related to lipid hydroperoxide concentration (see Chapter 4, this volume; [70]) and the relative amounts of LDL subtypes [71].

The inhibitory constituents of oLDL

The complexity of oLDL mentioned previously will give rise to a variety of oxidative products [51,72]. The major products of oxidative modification of LDL are hydroxy and hydroperoxy fatty acids, lysophosphatidylcholine, oxysterols, malondialdehyde and hydroxynonenal derivatives of the apolipoproteins [72]. In addition, peroxyl and hydroxyl radicals, superoxide anions, peroxynitrite, singlet oxygen and hydrogen peroxide are among the many possible agents that may be generated during the exposure of cells to lipoproteins [73].

        Several studies have sought to identify the inhibitory constituent(s) of oLDL that impair NO responses. In contrast to native LDL, the inhibition by oLDL requires a preincubation period, suggesting that lipophilic constituents are implicated [55,56], and this is further supported by evidence that the inhibitors are present in the lipid extract of oLDL [60]. Lysophosphatidylcholine is likely to be one of the inhibitory factors [56,60,61,69]. This may occur by action on the pathway for calcium mobilization (see Conclusions) or by inhibition of soluble guanylate cyclase [69]. However, the failure to find a positive correlation between inhibition of relaxation by oLDL and the lysophospholipid content suggests that other constituents of oLDL may contribute to the inhibition [56]. The hydroxy and hydroperoxy acids, 13-HODE, 15-HODE, 13-HPODE, 15-HETE and HPETE [64,74] (Fig. 3), which are produced by lipid peroxidation of LDL,

Fig. 3 The reversible inhibition of NO-dependent relaxations by 15-HPETE

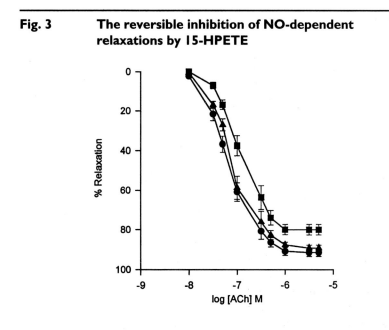

Precontracted aortic rings were relaxed in the presence and absence of 15-HPETE (15-hydroperoxyeicosatetraenoic acid) by cumulative doses of ACh [74]. ●, Control; ■, 15-HPETE (5 μM); ▲, washout.

also cause a small reversible inhibition of relaxation. This inhibition is mediated by activation of protein kinase C [64], a pathway known to inhibit NO responses [75]. In addition, 15-HETE and 15-HPETE directly contract vascular smooth muscle [74]. The fact that both HDL and serum albumin prevent the inhibition by oLDL [56] and lysophosphatidylcholine [69], but have no inhibitory action themselves, is further evidence in support of a lipophilic factor that translocates from the oLDL particles to the endothelial cells. Matsuda *et al.* [76], using radiolabelled lysophosphatidylcholine-loaded oLDL, confirmed that it was transferred to HDL and endothelial cells, although the participation of other lipid components in the inhibition is not excluded. Another study suggests that the uptake of the inhibitory components is via oLDL binding to scavenger receptors on endothelial cells. This requires confirmation using an antagonist besides dextran sulphate [66].

Alterations in the contractility during the development of atherosclerosis

Numerous studies show an enhancement in sensitivity to contractile agents during the development of atherosclerosis [12]. Angiographic studies of human coronary arteries of patients with coronary heart disease show a contraction to ACh and 5-HT, whereas the coronary vessels of the normal heart exhibit a vasodilatation (see section entitled Clinical studies). Similarly, isolated arteries from hypercholesterolaemic primates [77] exhibit hypercontractility to phenylephrine but become normal after the onset of atherosclerosis, whereas the contractile response to 5-HT is enhanced. A selective enhancement of 5-HT and a hyporesponsiveness to noradrenaline have also been described in cholesterol-fed New Zealand White rabbits [21] and Watanabe hereditary hyperlipidaemic rabbits at the early stages of atherosclerosis [25], but a more general effect was found in other studies [78]. These alterations in contractility are mimicked by exposure of rabbit aorta to oLDL [78,79] and are mediated via an increase in calcium influx [80] and stimulation of the phospholipase C–phosphoinositol pathway [81]. HETE and HPETE, oxidative products present in oxidatively modified LDL, induce contractions of rabbit aorta [74]. Expression and release of the vasoconstrictor peptide, endothelin is also enhanced by oLDL [82,83], which is consistent with the elevation of plasma endothelin levels during vasospastic angina [84]. Although impairment of vasodilatation contributes to the overall hyper-responsiveness in human atherosclerotic arteries, a major cause appears to be the increase in responsiveness of the vascular smooth muscle [78,79].

PGI$_2$ and vascular reactivity

General
Although PGI$_2$ is not thought to be the primary mediator of endothelium-dependent relaxation, it is important to realize that it prevents platelet activation and the release of many compounds which influence vascular reactivity. For example, thromboxane A$_2$ and high concentrations of 5-HT may cause vasoconstriction, which in normal arteries are overcome by the endothelium-

dependent relaxation produced by a combination of adenine nucleotides and 5-HT (in coronary vessels) released from platelets [85]. Hypercholesterolaemia will impair the latter response, causing vasoconstriction [85]. Furthermore, the indirect effect of lipoproteins on PGI_2 synthesis will further modify the responses of the platelets.

Effects of lipoproteins on PGI_2 synthesis

The effects of lipoproteins on the endothelium are less clear. Earlier reports suggested that LDL actually inhibits PGI_2 synthesis, whereas HDL stimulated it [86]. This fitted in well with early observations by Ross and Harker [87] of focal losses of endothelial cells in hypercholesterolaemia and a shortened platelet survival time. However, all recent studies have shown an increase in PGI_2 release in the presence of LDL, although less than that induced by the presence of HDL [88,89]. oLDL was found to increase the synthesis of PGI_2 by endothelial cells to a greater extent than native LDL [90]. There is little cross-reactivity with the PGI_2 metabolite, 6-ketoPGF$_{1\alpha}$ and oxidation products of LDL [91]: this was important because radioimmunoassays were used to determine PGI_2 release. It seems, therefore, that LDL increases rather than decreases PGI_2 synthesis and may be enhanced by lipoprotein oxidation which mobilizes intracellular calcium [80], a process which may accelerate the hydrolysis of phospholipids and the release of arachidonic acid. Further experimentation is required to study the time-course of these events and whether continued stimulation of the endothelium will ultimately lead to an impairment of PGI_2 synthesis. It is likely that this response is a protective action of the endothelium to prevent thrombus formation.

A role for native LDL has been proposed as a source of arachidonic acid for prostaglandin biosynthesis in endothelial cells [92] and resting monocytes [93]. This was based on the observation that in LDL receptor-negative cells from patients with homozygous hypercholesterolaemia, the biosynthesis of prostaglandins is less than those of the normal cells in the presence of LDL. However, it is known that the oxidation product of linoleic acid, 13-octadecadienoic acid, and its hydroperoxide increase PGI_2 synthesis [94], possibly through an increase in intracellular calcium. Cumene hydroperoxide appears to a have a similar effect [95], although lysolecithin decreases PGI_2 synthesis [96]. The action of radical species from cigarette smoke clearly inhibits PGI_2 synthesis [97].

The effects of lipoproteins on platelets

There has been extensive literature written on the effects of lipoproteins on platelets which now suggests that mildly oxidized LDLs may enhance their activation [98]. A number of reports have suggested that there is an effect of LDL on the inhibition of platelets by PGI_2. The inhibitory action of PGI_2 is impaired in platelets from patients with hypercholesterolaemia [99], which leads to a reduced accumulation of cyclic AMP in cells exposed to PGI_2. The dose of PGI_2 required to inhibit aggregation of isolated platelets is increased in the presence of LDL [100]. The decreased sensitivity to PGI_2 was also observed in patients with hypertriglyceridaemia [101]. More recently, it has been shown that both PGI_2- and adenosine-induced inhibition of platelet aggregation by ADP is decreased in familial hypercholesterolaemia [102]. A reduction in sensitivity to PGI_2 has been observed in patients with angina pectoris [103]. The responsiveness to PGI_2 was improved with exercise of the patients, an observation made earlier through training of healthy individuals [104]. The effects of lipoproteins on the sensitivity of platelets to NO have not been reported, but preliminary studies indicate that this too is impaired, although to a lesser extent (K.R. Bruckdorfer and K.M. Naseem, unpublished work).

Conclusions

The spectrum of changes in vascular reactivity observed in human and experimental models of hypercholesterolaemia is largely exhibited in normal arteries after acute exposure to LDL and oLDL. Although detailed differences in these lipoprotein studies are found between laboratories, they encompass the variations found in experimental models of atherosclerosis. There is a consensus of opinion that arteries become hypersensitive to vasoconstrictors, particularly 5-HT, and endothelium-dependent relaxation is impaired. The role of oLDL in these dysfunctions is summarized in Fig. 4(a).

An overall picture has emerged of the progression of the impairment of endothelium-dependent relaxation during the development of atherosclerosis. At the earliest stage, the dysfunction may be caused by defects in receptor-signal transduction [22], but as the disease progresses endothelium-dependent relaxation in general is affected and ultimately endothelium-independent vasodilatation is inhibited. In both experimental models and human studies, the dysfunction in endothelium-dependent relaxation in hypercholesterolaemia can be corrected by L-arginine [35–37], implying a decrease in NO synthesis due to a deficit in L-arginine. However, the high concentration of intracellular L-arginine found even after depriving endothelial cells of L-arginine for 24 h is sufficient to saturate NOS, which may suggest that L-arginine is compartmentalized [105–107]. The reversal of the impairment by L-arginine is likely to occur through increased NO synthesis by the iNOS isoform, which may be induced by cytokines released during the development of atherosclerosis, and possibly by oLDL (Fig. 4b). In addition, the upregulation of other isoforms of NOS may account for the increased synthesis observed by Minor et al. [34]. This view is supported by the finding of multiple isoforms, including iNOS in the blood vessel wall particularly in inflammatory cells during the development of human atherosclerosis [108].

Fig. 4   Impairment of vasodilatation in atherosclerotic arteries

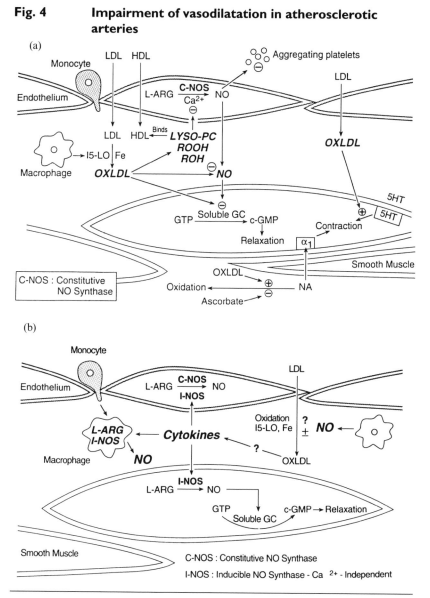

(a) Vasoactive effects of oxidized LDL; (b) possible role of iNOS. Abbreviations used: c-GMP, cyclic GMP; C-NOS, constitutive NO synthase; GC, guanylate cyclase; I-NOS, inducible NO synthase; L-ARG, L-arginine; 15-LO, 15-lipoxygenase; LYSO-PC, lysophosphatidylcholine; NA, noradrenaline; OXLDL, oxidized LDL; ROH, lipid hydroxy acids; ROOH, lipid hydroperoxy acids.

Other studies indicate that the dysfunction in endothelial-dependent relaxation is distal to synthesis and involves inactivation of the increased NO by an excess of superoxide anions and possibly other free radicals [33,34,44]. The inactivation may be caused partly by the continuous oxidative modification of LDL and its stimulation of superoxide anion formation [44,109] by the activation of protein kinase C [110], as well as by the release of superoxide anions from macrophages. Oxidative products in oLDL, such as lysophosphatidylcholine, hydroxy and hydroperoxy fatty acids, will also translocate to endothelial cells to inhibit calcium-dependent synthesis of NO by NOS (Fig. 4a) via activation of protein kinase C [111,112] and inhibition of calcium mobilization [112,113].

The endothelium may be the most important location of the effects of lipoproteins on platelet responsiveness. In turn, they may influence any stimulatory action of platelet secretory products on the endothelium. The effects on PGI_2 may appear anomalous, in that LDL reduces the sensitivity of platelets to the inhibitory effects of this prostaglandin, but at the endothelial level the lipoproteins appear to enhance its synthesis. Nevertheless, the apparent increase in PGI_2 and NO synthesis may be a protective response of the damaged endothelium designed to prevent local thrombus formation.

References

1. Moncada, S., Palmer, R.M.J. and Higgs, E.A. (1991) Pharmacol. Rev. **43**, 109–142
2. Vane, J.R., Anggard., E. and Botting, R.M. (1990) N. Engl. J. Med. **323**, 27–36
3. Cooke, J.P., Rossitch, E., Jr, Andon, N.A., Localzo, J. and Dzau, V.J. (1991) J. Clin. Invest. **88**, 1663–1671
4. Frangos, J.A., Eskin, S.G., McIntire, L.V. and Ives, C.L. (1984) Science **227**, 1477–1479
5. Holz, J., Forstermann, U., Pohl, U., Giesler, M. and Bassenge, E. (1984) J. Cardiovasc. Pharmacol. **6**, 1161–1169
6. Randall, M.D. and Griffiths, T.E. (1992) Am. J. Physiol. **263**, H752–H760
7. Stuehr, D.J. and Marletta, M.A. (1985) Proc. Natl. Acad. Sci. U.S.A. **82**, 7738–7742
8. Cho, HJ., Xie, Q.-W., Calaycay, J., Mumford, R.A., Swiderek, K.M., Lee, T.D. and Nathan, C. (1992) J. Exp. Med. **176**, 599–604
9. Fleming, I.G., Gray, G.A. and Stoclet, J.-C. (1991) Eur. J. Pharmacol. **200**, 375–376
10. Nishida, K., Harrison, D.G., Navas, J.P., Fisher, A.A. and Dockery S.P. (1992) J. Clin. Invest. **90**, 2092–2096
11. Furchgott, R.F. and Zawadzki, J.V. (1980) Nature (London) **288**, 373–376
12. Henderson, A.H. (1991) Br. Heart J. **65**, 116–125
13. Vita, J.A., Treasure, C.B., Nabel, M.D, McLenachan, J.M., Fish, R.D., Yeung, A.C., Vekshtein, V.I., Selwyn, A.P. and Ganz, P. (1990) Circulation **81**, 491–497
14. Werns, S.W., Joseph, A., Walton, J.A., Hsia, H.H., Nabel, E.G., Sanz, M.L. and Pitt, B. (1989) Circulation **79**, 287–294
15. Zeiher A.M., Drexler, H., Wollschlager, H. and Just, H. (1991) Circulation **83**, 391–401
16. Zeiher A.M., Drexler, H., Saubier, B. and Just, H. (1993) J. Clin. Invest. **92**, 652–662
17. Cox, D.A., Vita, J.A., Treasure, C.B., Fish, D., Alexander, R.W., Ganz, P. and Selwyn, A.P. (1989) Circulation **80**, 458–469
18. Drexler, H.A., Zeiher, A.M., Wollschlager, H., Meinertz, T., Just, H. and Bonzel, T. (1989) Circulation **80**, 466–474
19. Harrison, D.G., Freiman, P.C., Armstrong, M.L., Marcus, M.L. and Heistad, D.D. (1987) Circ. Res. **61** (Suppl. II), II-74–II-80
20. Cohen, R.A., Zitnay, K.M., Haudenschild, C.C. and Cunningham, L.D. (1988) Circ. Res. **63**,

903–910
21. Verbeuren, T.J. Jordaens, F.H., Zonnekeyn, L.L., Van Hove, C.E., Coene, M.-C. and Herman, A.G. (1986) Circ. Res. **58**, 552–564
22. Flavahan, N.A. (1992) Circulation **85**, 1927–1938
23. Galle, J., Busse, R. and Bassenge, E. (1991) Arteriosclerosis **11**, 1712–1718
24. Chinellato, A., Banchieri, L., Pandolfol, L., Ragazzi, E., Froldi, G., Nondo, F., Caparrotta, L. and Fassina, G. (1991) Atherosclerosis **89**, 223–230
25. Wines, P.A., Schmitz, J.M., Pfister, S.L., Clubb, F.J., Buja, L.M., Willerson, J.T. and Campbell, W.B. (1989) Arteriosclerosis **9**, 195–202
26. Chowienczyk, P.J., Watts, G.F., Cockcroft, J.R. Ritter, J.M. (1992) Lancet **340**, 1430–1432
27. Osborne, J.A., Siegman, M.J., Sedar, A.W., Mooers, S.U. and Lefer, A.M. (1989) Am. J. Physiol. **256**, C591–C597
28. Yamamoto, H., Bosaller, C., Cartwright Jr, J. and Henry, P.D. (1988) J. Clin. Invest. **81**, 1752–1758
29. Selke, F.W., Armstrong, M.I. and Harrison, D.G. (1990) Circulation **81**, 1586–1593
30. Kuo, L., Davis, M.J., Cannon, M.S. and Chilian, W.M. (1992) Circ. Res. **70**, 465–476
31. Juergens, J.L. and Bernatz, J.L. (1980) in Peripheral Vascular Diseases (Juergens, J.L., Spitell, J.A. and Fairbairn, I.I., eds.), pp. 253–293, WB Saunders Co., Philadelphia
32. Randall, M.D. Smith, J.A. and Griffiths, T.M. (1993) Br. J. Pharmacol. **109**, 838–844
33. Verbeuren, T.J., Jordaens, F.H., van Hove, C.E., van Hoydonck, A.-E. and Herman, A.G. (1990) Eur. J. Pharmacol. **191**, 173–184
34. Minor, R.L., Jr, Myers, P.R., Guerra R., Jr, Bates, J.R. and Harrison, D.G. (1990) J. Clin. Invest. **86**, 2109–2116
35. Drexler, H., Zeiher, A.M., Meinzer, K. and Just, H. (1991) Lancet **338**, 1546–1550
36. Girerd, X.J., Hirsch, A.T., Cooke, J.P., Dzau, V.J. and Creager, M.A. (1990) Circ. Res. **67**, 1301–1303
37. Cooke, J.P., Anon, N.A., Girerd, X.J., Hirsch, A.T. and Creager, M.A. (1991) Circulation **83**, 1057–1062
38. Lang, D., Smith, J.A. and Lewis, M.J. (1993) Br. J. Pharmacol. **108**, 290–292
39. Pomerantz, K.B., Hajjar, D.P., Levi, R. and Gross, S.S. (1993) Biochem. Biophys. Res. Commun. **191,** 103–109
40. Mugge, A. and Harrison, D.G. (1991) Blood Vesssels **28**, 354–357
41. Assreuy, J., Cunha, F.A., Liew, F.Y. and Moncada, S. (1993) Br. J. Pharmacol. **108**, 833–837
42. Waldman, S.A., Rappoport, R.M., Ginsburg, R. and Murad, F. (1986) Biochem. Pharmacol. **35**, 3525–3531
43. Jorens, P.G., Rosseneu, M., Devreese, A.-M., Bult, H., Maresceau, B. and Herman, A.G. (1992) Eur J. Pharmacol. **212**, 113–115
44. Ohara, Y., Peterson, T.E. and Harrison, D.G. (1993) J. Clin. Invest. **91**, 2546–2551
45. Mugge, A., Elwell, J.H., Peterson, T.E., Hofmeyer, T.G., Heistad, D.D. and Harrison, D.G. (1991) Circ. Res. **69**, 1293–1300
46. Nievelstein, P.E.M., Fogelman, A., Mottino, G. and Frank, J.S. (1991) **11**, 1795–1805
47. Zeiher, A.M., Schachinger, V. and Saurbier, B. (1993) Endothelium **1** (Suppl.), S89
48. Osborne, J.A., Lento, P.H., Siegfried, M.R., Stahl, G.L., Fusman, B. and Lefer, A.M. (1989) J. Clin. Invest. **83**, 465–475
49. Stewart-Lee, A.L., Forster, L.A., Nourooz-Zadeh, J. and Angaard, E.E. (1994) Arteriosclerosis Thrombosis **14 (3)**, 494–499
50. Simon, B.C., Haudenschild, C.C. and Cohen, R.A. (1993) J. Cardiovasc. Pharmacol. **21**, 893–901
51. Esterbauer, H., Dieber-Rothender, M., Waeg, G., Striegl, G. and Jurgens, G. (1990) Chem. Res. Toxicol. **3**, 77–92
52. Rosenfeld, M.E. (1991) Circulation **83**, 2137–2140
53. Andrews, H.E., Bruckdorfer, K.R., Dunn, R.C. and Jacobs, M. (1987) Nature (London) **327**, 237–239
54. Plane, F., Bruckdorfer, K.R. and Jacobs, M. (1989) Br. J. Pharmacol. **98**, 622P
55. Jacobs, M., Plane, F. and Bruckdorfer, K.R. (1990) Br. J. Pharmacol. **100**, 21–26
56. Plane, F., Bruckdorfer, K.R., Kerr, P., Steuer, A. and Jacobs, M. (1992) Br. J. Pharmacol. **105**, 216–222

57. Plane, F., Jacobs, M., McManus, D. and Bruckdorfer, K.R. (1993) Atherosclerosis **103**, 73–79
58. Galle, J., Mulsch, A., Busse, R. and Bassenge, E. (1991) Arteriosclerosis Thrombosis **11**, 198–203
59. Tomita, T, Ezaki, M., Miwa, M., Nakamura, K. and Inoue, Y. (1990) Circ. Res. **66**, 18–27
60. Kugiyama, K., Kerns, S.A., Morrisett, J.D., Roberts, R. and Henry, P.D. (1990) Nature (London) **344**, 160–162
61. Yokoyama, M., Hirata, K., Miyake, R., Akita, H., Ishikawa, Y. and Fukuzaki, H. (1990) Biophys. Biochem. Res. Commun. **168**, 301–308
62. Simon, B.C., Cunningham, L.D. and Cohen, R.A. (1990) J. Clin. Invest. **86**, 75–79
63. Thomas, C.E. and Jackson, R.L. (1991) J. Pharmacol. Exp. Ther. **256**, 1182–1188
64. Buckley, C., McManus, D., Bruckdorfer, K.R. and Jacobs, M. (1994) Br. J. Pharmacol. **112**, 222P
65. Buckley, C., Bund, S., McTaggart, F., Bruckdorfer, K.R., Jacobs, M. and Oldham, A. (1993) Br. J. Pharmacol. **110**, 85P
66. Tanner, F.C., Noll, G., Boulanger, C.M. and Luscher, M.D. (1991) Circulation **83**, 2012–2020
67. Kerr, P. and Jacobs, M. (1992) in The Biology of Nitric Oxide: Part 1, Physiological and Clinical Aspects (Moncada, S., Marletta, M.A., Hibbs, J.B. Jr., and Higgs, E.A., eds.), pp. 193–195, Portland Press, London
68. Chin, J.A., Azhar, S. and Hofman, B.B. (1992) J. Clin. Invest. **89**, 10–18
69. Schmidt, K., Klatt, P., Graier, W.F., Kostner, G.M., and Kukovetz, W.R. (1990) Biochem. Biophys. Res. Commun. **2**, 614–619
70. O'Leary, V.J., Darley-Usmar, V.M., Russell, L.J., Stone, D. (1992) Biochem. J. **282**, 631–634
71. De Graaf, J., Heidi, L.M., Hak-Lemmers, H.L., Hectors, M.P.C., Demacker, P.N.M., Hendriks, J.C.M. and Stalenhoef, A.F.H. (1991) Arteriosclerosis **11**, 298–306
72. Bruckdorfer, K.R. (1990) Curr. Opin. Lipidol. **1**, 529–535
73. Bruckdorfer, K.R. (1993) Curr. Opin. Lipidol. **4**, 238–243
74. Buckley, C., McManus, D., Bruckdorfer, K.R. and Jacobs, M. (1994) Br. J. Pharmacol. **112**, 539P
75. Smith, J.A. and Lang, D. (1990) Br. J. Pharmacol. **99**, 565–572
76. Matsuda, Y., Hirata, K., Inoue, N., Suematsu, M., Kawashima, S., Akita, H. and Yokoyama, M. (1993) Circ. Res. **72**, 1103–1109
77. Lopez, J.A., Armstrong, M.L., Pregors, D.J. and Heistad, D.D. (1989) Circulation **79**, 698–705
78. Galle, J., Bassenge, E. and Busse, R. (1990) Circ. Res. **66**, 1287–1293
79. Plane, F., Bruckdorfer, K.R., Jacobs, M. (1990) Br. J. Pharmacol. **99**, 220P
80. Galle, J., Luckhoff, A., Busse, R., Bassenge, E. (1990) Eicosanoids **3**, 81–86
81. Resink, T.J. (1992) Arteriosclerosis Thrombosis **12**, 278–285
82. Asano, M. and Hidaka, H. (1979) J. Pharmacol. Exp. Ther. **208**, 347–353
82. Martin-Nizard, F., Houssaini, H.S., Debattre, S.L., Duriez, P. and Fruchart, J.-C. (1993) FEBS Lett. **293**, 127–130
83. Boulanger, C.M., Tanner, F.C., Bea, M.L., Hahn, A.W., Werner, A. and Luscher, T. (1992) Circ. Res. **83**, 1191–1197
84. Toyo-oka, T., Aizawa, T., Suziki, N., Hirata, Y., Miyauchi, T., Shun, W.S., Yanagisawa, M., Masaki, T. and Sugimoto, T. (1991) Circulation **83**, 476–483
85. Vanhoutte, P.M. (1991) Eur. Heart J. **12** (Suppl. E), 25–32
86. Fleisher, L.N., Tall, A.R., Witt, L.D., Miller, R.W. and Cannon, P.J. (1982) J. Biol. Chem. **257**, 6653–6655
87. Ross, R. and Harker, L. (1976) Science **193**, 1094–1100
88. Spector, A.A., Scanu, A.M., Kaduce, T.L., Figard, P.H., Fless, G.M. and Czervionke, R.L. (1985) J. Lipid Res. **26**, 288–297
89. Spector, A.A. (1988) Semin. Thromb. Haemostasis **14**, 196–201
90. Triau, J.E., Meydani, S.N. and Schaefer, E.J. (1988) Arteriosclerosis Thrombosis **8**, 810–818
91. Zhang, H., Davis, W.B., Chen, X., Whisler, R.L. and Cornwell, D.G. (1989) J. Lipid Res. **30**, 141–148

92. Habenicht, A.J., Salbach, P., Goerig, M., Zeh, W., Janssen Timmen, U., Blattner, C., King, W.C. and Glomset, J.A. (1990) Prostaglandins Med. 5, 451–467
93. Salbach, P.B., Specht, E., Vonhodenberg, E., Kossmann, J., Janssentimmen, U., Schneider, W.J., Hugger, P., King, W.C., Glomset, J.A. and Habenicht, A.J.R. (1992) Proc. Natl. Acad. Sci. U.S.A. 89, 2439–2443
94. Demeyer, G.R.Y., Bult, H., Verbeuren, T.J. and Herman, A.G. (1992) Br. J. Pharmacol. 107, 597–603
95. Griesmacher, A., Weigel, G., David, M., Schimke, I. and Mueller, M.M. (1992) Thromb. Res. 65, 721–731
96. Stoll, L.L., Oskarsson, H.J. and Spector, A.A. (1992) Am. J. Physiol. 262, H1853–H1860
97. Jeremy, J. and Mikhailidis, D.P. (1990) J. Smok. Rel. Dis. 1, 59–69
98. Bruckdorfer, K.R. (1992) Atherosclerosis IX: Proceedings of the Ninth International Symposium in Atherosclerosis: Chicago (Stein, O. Eisenberg, S. and Stein, Y., eds.), R and L Creative Communications Ltd, Tel Aviv
99. Colli, S., Lombroso, M., Maderna, P., Tremoli, E. and Nicosia, S. (1983) Biochem. Pharmacol. 32, 1989–1993
100. Bruckdorfer, K.R., Buckley, S. and Hassall, D.G. (1984) Biochem. J. 233, 189–196
101. Curtis, L.D., Jones, R.J., Machin, S.J. and Betteridge, D.J. (1984) Eur. J. Clin. Invest. 14, 37
102. Gasser, J.A., McCarthy, S.N., Jay, R.H. and Betteridge, D.J. (1989) Atherosclerosis 79, 95
103. Kishi, Y., Ashikaga, T. and Numano, F. (1992) Am. Heart J. 123, 291–297
104. Dix, C.J., Hassall, D.G. and Bruckdorfer, K.R. (1985) Thromb. Haemostasis 51, 385–387
105. Mayer, B., Schmidt, K., Humbert, P. and Bohme, E. (1989) Biochem. Biophys. Res. Commun. 164, 678–685
106. Baydoun, A.R., Emery, P., Pearson, J.D. and Mann, G.E. (1990) Biochem. Biophys. Res. Commun. 173, 940–948
107. Mitchell, J., Hecker, M., Angaard, E.E. and Vane, J. (1990) Eur. J. Pharmacol. 182, 572–576
108. Wilcox, J.X., Subramanian, R., Ross, C.E., Tracey, W.R., Pollock, J.S., Harrison, D.G. and Marsden, P.A. (1994) Circulation 90, 1–298
109. Tagawa, H., Tomoike, H. and Nakamura, M. (1991) Circ. Res. 68, 330–337
110. Lehr, H.A., Becker, M., Marklund, S.L., Hubner, C., Arfors, K.E., Kohlschutter, A. and Messmer, K. Arteriosclerosis Thrombosis 12, 824–829
111. Kugiyama, K., Ohgushi, M., Sugiyama, S., Murohara, T., Fukunaga, A.K., Miyamoto, E. and Yasue, H. (1992) Circ. Res. 71, 1422–1428
112. Inoue, N., Hirata, K.-I., Yamada, M., Hamamori, Y., Matsuda, Y., Akita, H. and Yokoyama, M. (1992) Circ. Res. 71, 1410–1421
113. Elliot, S.J. and Doan, T.N. (1993) Biochem. J. 292, 385–393

8

Free radicals and the inflammatory response

Kenneth S. Kilgore and Benedict R. Lucchesi*

Department of Pharmacology, University of Michigan Medical School, Ann Arbor, MI 48109-0626, U.S.A.

Introduction

The use of thrombolytic agents as therapy for the treatment of myocardial infarction has proved to be of benefit in decreasing patient mortality [1]. These agents, however, have revealed another aspect of myocardial infarction: the effects associated with reperfusion. It has been proposed that the rapid restoration of flow to an ischaemic area is associated with the extension of cellular injury. Thus, the very event that is essential for survival of the tissue, restoration of blood flow, may contribute to the extension of myocardial injury. The topic of reperfusion injury has received attention in an effort to determine its true significance and its underlying mechanisms. Through these efforts, a number of factors have been implicated, thereby allowing for the development of therapeutic agents to decrease the deleterious effects associated with reperfusion of previously ischaemic, but still viable, tissue.

There is controversy regarding the existence of reperfusion injury. It has been suggested that reperfusion accelerates evidence of irreversible cell injury so that changes characteristic of infarction become evident sooner or appear worse [2]. On the other hand, there are those who contend that reperfusion itself results in cellular damage not otherwise due to the ischaemic insult. Reperfusion injury represents a paradoxical increase in myocardial injury that would not occur in the absence of reflow. Reperfusion injury, therefore, is the conversion of myocytes from a reversibly injured state to that of irreversible injury; an event that can be attributed to reperfusion itself. This type of injury involves the death of myocytes that were not irreversibly injured before reperfusion and is characterized by definite ultrastructural alterations that differ substantially from those that occur as a result of ischaemic cell death. Ultrastructural changes with reperfusion involve myocyte disintegration with 'explosive' cell swelling, and fragmentation of mitochondria. Most notable

*To whom correspondence should be addressed.

is the appearance of contraction band necrosis due to the massive accumulation of intracellular calcium ion. Tissue injury due to ischaemia, without reperfusion, has the microscopic appearance of pale, relaxed myofibrils with preserved cell structure; commonly referred to as 'coagulation necrosis'.

Two factors implicated in the development of reperfusion injury, molecular oxygen and the inflammatory response, have been shown to be necessary for myocardial salvage [3]. Thus, a paradoxical situation develops where the very processes needed for survival of the tissue may in fact be detrimental. While there can be no debate regarding the importance of early reperfusion, the events associated with reperfusion must be taken into consideration. This discussion will focus on the current understanding regarding the respective roles of oxygen-derived free radicals and the inflammatory response in reperfusion injury. The two events are not mutually exclusive, but act in concert to extend the degree of tissue damage beyond that resulting from the ischaemic insult.

Oxygen-derived free radicals

Molecular oxygen, while essential for maintaining cell viability, is believed to be one of the primary factors involved in reperfusion injury. This represents the first paradox of reperfusion injury: oxygen, when metabolized to a reactive radical, may be detrimental to the tissue. One of the early indications that molecular oxygen was involved in the development of reperfusion injury was the observation that perfusion of the hypoxic heart with an oxygenated solution enhanced myocardial injury, while a solution devoid of oxygen (hypoxic reperfusion) did not increase the extent of tissue injury [4]. Since this time, it has been apparent that the introduction of molecular oxygen to the ischaemic myocardium results in the formation of oxygen-derived free radicals [5,6]. These observations are supported by the use of electron-resonance spectroscopy and spin-trapping agents to detect free radicals in the ischaemic zone when perfusion with oxygenated medium is reintroduced to the ischaemic tissue [5,6]. Superoxide anion (O_2^-), hydrogen peroxide (H_2O_2) and the highly reactive hydroxyl radical ($OH^.$) are the most prominently mentioned free radicals in the pathogenesis of reperfusion injury.

A number of endogenous intracellular factors [superoxide dismutase (SOD), catalase, glutathione peroxidase] are present under normal conditions which serve to protect the myocardium against free radical-induced injury. During an ischaemic insult of sufficient duration and upon the subsequent reperfusion, however, it is speculated that the intracellular antioxidants may be limited and subsequently overwhelmed by the sudden generation of reactive oxygen metabolites [7]. Cytotoxic metabolites of oxygen can be derived from intracellular sources (e.g. mitochondrial metabolism) as well as from extracellular sources, of which the invading polymorphonuclear leucocyte (neutrophil) represents the most important mediator of oxidative injury, by virtue of its ability to give rise to a wide range of cytotoxic metabolites of oxygen [O_2^-, H_2O_2, OH^- and hypochlorous acid ($HOCl$)]. To supplement the naturally occurring defence mechanisms, inhibitors of free radical formation and scavengers of oxygen free radicals have been used in a number of experimental models, in an attempt to decrease tissue injury. The use of free radical scavengers has met with varying degrees of success. Jolly *et al.* [8] utilized the oxygen free radical scavenger SOD and the H_2O_2-degrading enzyme catalase to decrease myocardial infarct size in the canine heart. Other studies utilizing SOD alone and SOD conjugated to polyethylene glycol have obtained similar results [9,10]. However, a number of other investigators have failed to see protection with SOD [11,12]. Although the reasons for these discrepancies are not known, it has been speculated that the half-life of the SOD molecule (10 min) and the length of the ischaemic interval, plus the lack of a critical stenosis, may be responsible for the divergent results among the several laboratories.

Free radical-induced cellular injury

What makes a free radical a potent adversary is its ability to cross biological membranes and damage a number of cellular components. Thus, radicals generated in an environment where defence mechanisms have been impaired have the ability to inflict damage throughout the entire cell and surrounding tissue. Some of the primary targets of free radicals are the lipids and proteins that constitute the cell membrane [13]. Unsaturated lipids containing double bonds are vulnerable to peroxidation, resulting in the formation of lipid peroxides, aldehydes and lipid hydroperoxides [13]. The intermediates of lipid peroxidation have been shown to alter protein function through fragmentation or polymerization of proteins [14]. Thus, not only is membrane integrity compromised, but the products of the reactions may be cytotoxic. In addition to lipids, both membrane-bound and intracellular proteins are vulnerable to free radical attack. By denaturing proteins, a number of cellular functions, including intracellular transport and metabolism, are altered. The ability of free radicals to oxidize sulphydryl groups on methionine residues allows for proteins to be altered in a number of different ways, including conformational changes, denaturation and enhanced susceptibility to hydrolysis [15,16]. Amino acids such as tyrosine, proline, tryptophan and phenylalanine are oxidized by free radicals. Membrane proteins that serve enzymic or receptor functions would be vulnerable to modification by free radicals, thereby impairing important cellular and membrane functions [17].

Origins of free radical generation

The potential origins of free radical generation are varied, ranging from extracellular sources to a number of intracellular organelles. Induction of the inflammatory response may bring neutrophils and monocytes into the reperfused area. Both phagocytic cell types have been shown to react with products of oxygen, including: O_2^-, OH$^.$, H_2O_2 and HOCl. The vascular endothelium has been implicated in the production of oxygen radicals. The endothelial enzyme xanthine oxidase (derived from the conversion of xanthine dehydrogenase), is thought to produce O_2^- and H_2O_2 through the utilization of hypoxanthine as a substrate [18]. Experimental evidence for the role of xanthine oxidase in reperfusion injury is derived from studies suggesting that allopurinol, an inhibitor of the enzyme, affords protection to the myocardium subjected to regional ischaemia and reperfusion [19]. Despite the positive outcome with the use of allopurinol, the drug was effective only if administered 24 h before the ischaemic insult. The results suggest that a metabolite of allopurinol, most probably oxypurinol, was responsible for the observed protective effect [19]. However, the study cited was conducted in the dog, where xanthine oxidase is known to be present. In other species, including rabbit and human, both xanthine dehydrogenase and xanthine oxidase are absent from the myocardium and may be confined to the endothelial cell. The variability among species in the activity of xanthine oxidase in myocardial tissue has led to doubt that this is the predominant route of radical production in humans [20,21]. Furthermore, the study by Werns et al. [22], using the highly effective inhibitor of xanthine oxidase, amflutazole, failed to show cardioprotection despite the fact that the enzyme was inhibited as shown by the decrease in uric acid in the coronary sinus blood of treated animals.

Organelles, including cellular membranes and mitochondria, provide an additional source of free radicals. Membrane biosynthesis of arachidonic acid metabolites by cyclo-oxygenase and lipoxygenase pathways has been shown to result in H_2O_2 and O_2^- formation [23]. Mitochondria normally produce H_2O_2 through the electron-transport chain. It is plausible that production is increased during ischaemia or the ability to reduce H_2O_2 to OH$^.$, and then to H_2O, is lost [18]. The latter explanation is supported by the observation that endogenous cellular constituents — such as glutathione, glutathione peroxidase and SOD — which serve to protect the tissue from free radical attack are depleted during the ischaemic insult and are not available to defend the cell against the anticipated increase in free radical production associated with the reintroduction of molecular oxygen during myocardial reperfusion [24].

Neutrophil-mediated myocardial injury

The neutrophil is one of the primary components of the inflammatory system implicated in reperfusion injury. These cells possess the capacity to impose cellular injury through a number of mechanisms. Although the primary function of the neutrophil is to defend the host from microbial invasion, it is appreciated that neutrophils exert a detrimental effect in ischaemia–reperfusion injury. The neutrophils begin to infiltrate into the jeopardized myocardial region within 60 min after the onset of ischaemia and continue to accumulate for up to 24 h [25]. Histological observations have shown a direct relationship between the duration of ischaemia and the extent of neutrophil infiltration, and infarct size has been shown to be proportional to the number of accumulated neutrophils [26–28]. More substantial evidence is derived from a number of studies utilizing experimental animals that have been depleted of circulating neutrophils. The use of filters [29], cytotoxic agents [30] and neutrophil antisera [27], in addition to inhibiting neutrophil adhesion [31], has been shown to decrease ultimate infarct size, an effect related to decreased neutrophil accumulation.

Adhesion of neutrophils to the endothelium

Adherence of the neutrophil to the endothelium is a critical event in the evolution of reperfusion injury. Simpson *et al.* utilized an anti-CD11b (MO1) antibody to reduce infarct size in the canine myocardium. The anti-MO1 anti-body was administered 45 min before the induction of regional myocardial ischaemia. After reperfusion, infarct size was found to decrease by 46%. Inhibition of neutrophil infiltration was associated with this decreased infarct size. The use of antibodies directed against the CD11b component of the het-erodimeric neutrophil-adhesion-promoting receptor may decrease neutrophil adhesion by inhibiting the interaction of MO1 with intracellular adhesion mol-ecule-1 (ICAM-1), or inhibiting the interaction of the neutrophil with iC3b-opsonized particles. Monoclonal antibodies directed against the CD18 epitope of the CD11/CD18 adhesion complex has also afforded protection after regional ischaemia–reperfusion in the rabbit [32]. These and other studies indicate that before neutrophils can elicit cellular damage, they must first adhere to the endothelium and/or myocytes in the jeopardized region that has been subjected to ischaemic injury and reperfusion. Once firmly attached to the endothelial cell, the neutrophil may migrate through the endothelial layer, thus gaining access to the surrounding myocardial tissue. The accumulation of inflammatory cells, along with their potential to form cytotoxic oxygen metabolites and release proteolytic enzymes, establishes the proper environ-ment for expansion of the area of tissue injury beyond that irreversibly injured by the ischaemic insult.

The mechanisms of neutrophil adherence are complex, involving a number of different adhesion molecules on both the neutrophil and endothe-lial cell. Both neutrophils and endothelial cells constitutively express adhesion molecules on their respective membranes. However, in response to the appro-priate stimuli, a series of events is set in motion that initiates cell–cell interac-tions leading to rapid neutrophil adherence, transmigration, accumulation in the interstitial space and neutrophil activation.

Neutrophil adhesion: the early events

Two events, 'rolling' of the neutrophil along the endothelium and 'tethering' of the neutrophil to the endothelial cell, may be associated with the early cell–cell interactions leading to neutrophil–endothelial cell adherence. Studies with the use of intravital microscopy have demonstrated that before firm adhesion is established, the neutrophil 'rolls' along the endothelium at a rate 100 times slower than the flow of blood [33]. This event is mediated, in part, by the neutrophil glycoprotein L-selectin, a member of the selectin family of adhesion molecules [33,34]. The endothelial counter-receptor for L-selectin has yet to be determined, although N-linked or O-linked sugars on endothelial cells have been mentioned to serve in this capacity [35]. In response to stimulation of the neutrophil by different cytokines, L-selectin is shed rapidly from the neutrophil surface. The 'shedding' of the molecule is actually a proteolytic cleavage near the transmembrane domain [36,37]. As will be discussed in more detail, this cleavage coincides with the upregulation of another adhesion molecule, the CD11b/CD18 complex [38]. Although the importance of rolling is not entirely clear, it has been suggested that this process allows for the initial binding of the neutrophil to the endothelial cell and places the neutrophil in close proximity to the endothelial surface, thereby facilitating the subsequent event needed for securing intimate cell–cell contact.

P-selectin (PADGEM, GMP-140) is stored in Weibel–Palade bodies within the endothelial cell. Upon stimulation, these granules are translocated to the endothelial surface. Studies using thrombin and histamine to stimulate the endothelium have been shown to result in expression of P-selectin [39]. This expression is a transitory event, reaching a maximum within 15 min of stimulation, after which the molecule is again internalized [39]. Exposure to certain oxidants has been shown to enhance the exposure of P-selectin [40]. The conditions seen during reperfusion, therefore, may provide a greater means of interaction of the neutrophil with P-selectin. Like L-selectin, P-selectin may be involved in neutrophil rolling on the endothelial surface. In contrast to L-selectin, the primary role of P-selectin may be to 'tether' the neutrophil to the endothelium. The importance of P-selectin is demonstrated by the use of soluble P-selectin or by antibodies directed against the molecule to inhibit neutrophil adhesion. Mulligan et al. [41] have demonstrated that anti-P-selectin antibodies partially prevent pulmonary vascular injury in the rat after infusion of cobra venom factor. This study underscores the importance of P-selectin in the early events of neutrophil–endothelial cell adhesion.

Platelet activating factor (PAF) should also be mentioned when discussing the early events of neutrophil adhesion. PAF is a biologically active phospholipid not expressed under normal conditions, but is synthesized rapidly upon perturbation of the endothelial cell membrane. Unlike other cell types, endothelial cells do not release PAF into the fluid phase, but express it on the membrane surface [42]. PAF has the unique capacity to activate neutrophils and to stimulate surface expression of P-selectin. The importance of PAF in the sequence of neutrophil adhesion is best exemplified by the ability of PAF antagonists to decrease neutrophil adhesion [43].

The receptor on the surface of the neutrophil for PAF is a member of the G-protein family [44]. Activation of this receptor leads to upregulation of both CD11a/CD18 and CD11b/CD18. Thus, a principal role of this molecule is not only to adhere the neutrophil to the endothelium, but also to 'prime' the neutrophil to upregulate other adhesion receptors [45]. Upregulation of the β_2-integrins may not be the only effect that PAF has upon adhesion molecules. Fluid-phase PAF has been shown to elicit shedding of L-selectin [46]. Although it has not been shown conclusively, it is likely that membrane-bound PAF also has this effect. Lorant *et al.* [45] have proposed a juxtacrine interaction between PAF and P-selectin. In this scenario, P-selectin acts to tether the neutrophil to the endothelial cell, thereby allowing for interaction with PAF. This interaction provides an example of how different groups of adhesion molecules, as opposed to single receptor–ligand interactions, work in concert to regulate the early events associated with adhesion.

The β_2-integrins

After the early events of neutrophil adhesion, the neutrophil becomes attached to the endothelial cell by the CD11/CD18 β_2-integrins. While early adhesion to the endothelium is of short duration, attachment via the β_2-integrins is of a more firm and longer-lasting nature. The CD11/CD18 glycoproteins possess a common β-subunit (CD18) non-covalently bound to a distinct α-subunit, designated as either LFA-1 (CD11a), MO1 (CD11b, Mac-1) or gp150/95 (CD11c). Like P-selectin, MO1 is stored in intracellular sites and is mobilized to the cell surface in response to the appropriate stimuli (e.g. C5a). At the surface, the molecule serves as the receptor for complement-derived iC3b opsonized particles and is not only involved in adhesion, but also in chemotaxis and spreading of the neutrophil [47,48]. The importance of the MO1 subunit in mediating neutrophil adherence and reperfusion injury is seen in the ability of antibodies directed against MO1 to decrease the extent of ischaemia–reperfusion injury in the canine myocardium [31,49]. In addition to serving as the receptor for iC3b, MO1 interacts with ICAM-1 located on the endothelial surface. Endothelial cells in the basal state express low levels of ICAM-1. Stimulation by cytokines such as interleukin(IL)-1 and tumour necrosis factor (TNF) upregulates expression of ICAM-1, leading to upregulation of endothelial-leucocyte adhesion molecule-1, a member of the selectin family. The upregulation of these ligands is maximal within 4–6 h [50].

Antibodies to ICAM-1 not only decrease neutrophil adhesion, but reduce infarct size in the ischaemic–reperfused rabbit heart [32,51]. In summary, the sequence of events associated with adhesion involves a number of neutrophil–endothelial cell interactions that are expressed sequentially over the course of hours, ultimately culminating in the inflammatory response to injury. It is likely that the early events (first minutes) in neutrophil–endothelial cell adhesion are mediated through a transient interaction, via the selectins (L-selectin, P-selectin) and the phospholipid molecule, PAF. The β_2-integrins, especially MO1 and perhaps LFA-1, are responsible for adhesion lasting longer periods of time (minutes to hours). During this interval, the neutrophil may become firmly attached to the endothelium before moving out of the vasculature into the surrounding tissue. During chronic episodes of inflammation, the third member of the β_2-integrin family, GP150/95, is likely to become the primary mediator of neutrophil adhesion [52]. Expression of the neutrophil β_2-integrin, MO-1 (CD11b/CD18), is related to stimulation of the neutrophil by C5a and the endothelial cell ligand for MO-1 is iC3b. The inflammatory response to injury, therefore, involves activation of the complement system which is responsible, in part, for orchestrating the carefully timed sequence of events associated with the recruitment of neutrophils to the site of injury and, ultimately, repair of the damage.

Neutrophil-induced cellular injury

Activated neutrophils possess multiple mechanisms by which they contribute to the inflammatory response in the ischaemic/reperfused myocardium. Adhesion and subsequent migration out of the vascular bed are necessary events for the neutrophil to induce myocyte damage, a conclusion supported by evidence *in vitro* [53].

An important cytotoxic mechanism present in the neutrophil is the ability to mediate tissue damage through the formation and release of oxygen-derived free radical species. Stimulation of the neutrophil by a number of soluble factors, including complement-derived C5a, has been shown to result in a rapid increase in oxygen consumption. The intracellular metabolism of molecular oxygen leads to the formation of a number of toxic metabolites, including O_2^-, H_2O_2, $OH^{\cdot}$, HOCl and chloramine ($RNHCL^-$). Most of these radicals are in the form of O_2^-, which is enzymically converted to H_2O_2 through the action of SOD. In addition to its toxic effects by virtue of being converted to $OH^{\cdot}$, H_2O_2 may induce an increase in neutrophil adhesion. Gasic *et al.* [54] have shown that treatment of canine isolated blood vessels with H_2O_2 increased neutrophil adhesion through a CD18–PAF-dependent mechanism. This is supported by the observation that H_2O_2 increases PAF synthesis by human endothelial cells [55]. Thus, a positive feedback mechanism is established whereby activated neutrophils may recruit additional circulating neutrophils.

Neutrophils are capable of releasing a number of proteolytic enzymes that contribute to transmigration from the vascular bed and extend the area of tissue injury. Two proteases, collagenase and gelatinase, are activated by HOCl and are capable of directly lysing endothelial cells [56].

Furthermore, neutrophil-derived proteolytic enzymes are capable of degrading components of the extracellular matrix, including elastin, collagen and other cellular proteins [56]. In addition to their direct effects, the neutrophil-derived proteases exert indirect effects by acting on plasma proteins, leading to activation of the complement system and fibrin formation, and participating in the formation of plasma kinins [57]. Cationic proteins released in conjunction with the proteases have been found not only to affect clot formation, but to elicit release of vasoactive substances from mast cells, further aggravating the conditions found during evolution of an acute myocardial infarction. [58]. Thus, substances released from the neutrophil may not only inflict cellular damage, but may aid in migration of the neutrophil into the surrounding tissue. The role that proteases play in reperfusion injury has yet to be elucidated completely. Inhibitors of neutrophil proteolytic enzymes, such as aprotinin, have been shown to limit myocardial infarct size in the experimental animal, although the mechanism for this protection has not been substantiated [59,60]. However, Bolli *et al.* have found that the suppression of protease activity by a number of different inhibitors failed to decrease myocardial infarct size in experiments carried out in the rat [61,62].

It is conceivable that neutrophils remaining in the vasculature may have deleterious effects upon the myocardium. Since neutrophils have the ability to form aggregates, small capillaries may become physically obstructed or 'plugged'. This plugging has been suggested to account for the 'no-reflow' phenomenon, where areas of the ischaemic region are not properly reperfused [63]. Early evidence for this was seen by the ability of neutrophil depletion to reduce the development of the no-reflow phenomenon in skeletal muscle. Recently, Jerome *et al.* [64] have verified this observation by showing that the CD11/CD18 complex is important in the development of the no-reflow phenomenon. In addition, a correlation has been shown to exist between the number of neutrophils in the microvasculature and the severity of the no-reflow phenomenon. The actions of neutrophils upon the vasculature are not limited to the small postcapillary venules. Neutrophils may affect larger vessels such as arterioles and precapillary vessels. Release of vasoconstricting agents from activated neutrophils is thought to decrease vessel diameter, resulting in decreased perfusion of the surrounding tissue [65]. The decrease in perfusion may be exacerbated by release of factors from the neutrophil, such as PAF, which serves to activate circulating platelets. The accumulation of platelets would increase vascular plugging in addition to releasing platelet-derived products that act upon the vasculature, adding to the impairment of regional blood flow [65].

Formation and release of arachidonic acid metabolites from neutrophils participate in amplifying the inflammatory response. Among the most active of these metabolites are the leukotrienes, generated by the action of 5-lipoxygenase on arachidonic acid [66]. The most prominent leukotrienes are

LTA4, LTB4, LTC4 and LTD4, which function as mediators of the inflammatory response. Neutrophil-derived LTB4 functions as a potent stimulator of neutrophil aggregation and chemotaxis into the surrounding tissue, thereby serving to reinforce the development of the local inflammatory response. LTB4 has also been shown to increase the production of O_2^- and, to a lesser degree, stimulate the release of intracellular granules from the neutrophil [66, 67]. The tissue content of LTB4 is increased in the infarcted myocardium, suggesting a role for this eicosanoid in reperfusion injury [68]. Other metabolites, including LTC4 and LTD4, affect neutrophil function albeit in an indirect manner. Both of these metabolites have been shown to stimulate endothelial cells to produce PAF which, as discussed previously, may serve to stimulate neutrophils and promote adhesion [69]. In addition, these metabolites may further stimulate neutrophils by augmenting the actions of C5a. Both LTC4 and LTD4 increase vascular permeability and are potent vasoconstrictors. The vasoconstricting effect exacerbates the degree of the ischaemic injury. Thus, formation of arachidonic acid metabolites by neutrophils is part of a positive feedback mechanism serving to potentiate the inflammatory response within the ischaemic zone.

Chemotactic factors

An integral aspect of neutrophil-mediated damage is the recruitment of circulating neutrophils. To accomplish this task, mechanisms must exist by which circulating neutrophils are drawn to the ischaemic region. The ability to inhibit recruitment may provide a therapeutic avenue to inhibit neutrophil accumulation and is therefore the subject of intensive study.

The emigration of neutrophils is directed by the generation of a gradient of soluble factors released from several sources, including the endothelium and the neutrophil itself. However, this theory is called into question by a number of investigators who argue that activation of neutrophils by soluble factors would lead to the shedding of L-selectin and shape change by the neutrophil [37,38,46,70]. It has been shown that the loss of L-selectin before contact with the endothelium prevents the neutrophil from adhering to the endothelium [71]. Therefore, other mechanisms exist by which chemotactic factors recruit neutrophils to the site of injury. One suggestion is that the chemotactic gradient is not soluble, but bound to the surface of endothelial cells [72]. An example of this type of chemoattractant is PAF, which is expressed on the surface of stimulated endothelial cells. Another molecule synthesized by the endothelium, interleukin (IL)-8 [neutrophil attractant/activation protein 1 (MAP-1)], has received increased attention. Within 4–24 h after stimulation, endothelial cells begin to synthesize and release the IL-8 polypeptide [73–75]. Although initially released into the fluid phase, IL-8 has been shown to be ultimately deposited on the endothelial cell surface [76].

Binding of the neutrophil to IL-8 results in activation of a G-protein-coupled receptor, resulting in shedding of L-selectin and upregulation of the CD11/CD18 complex [77]. The advantage to this approach is that the neutrophil has established contact with the endothelium before shedding L-selectin and undergoing shape change. It has been suggested that the soluble form of IL-8 mediates neutrophil adhesion. Preincubation of neutrophils or endothelial cells with soluble IL-8 reduces neutrophil transmigration [78]. The mechanism of this desensitization is not known, although it has been suggested that down-regulation of L-selectin on the neutrophil surface may play a role. This point remains controversial and is in need of further examination.

The complement system, through the generation of the chemotactic factor C5a, serves a major role in attracting neutrophils to the site of tissue injury. The importance of the complement system in neutrophil recruitment is demonstrated by the observation that depletion of complement by cobra venom factor reduces neutrophil infiltration into the myocardium and has the overall effect of reducing myocardial injury associated with ischaemia–reperfusion. C5a and other complement-derived factors, including C3a and C4a, aid neutrophil infiltration into the myocardium by increasing vascular permeability and altering vascular tone. The membrane attack complex (MAC) of complement has been shown to increase the production of arachidonic acid metabolites, including the potent chemotactic factor LTB4 [79].

As stated previously, reperfusion of the ischaemic myocardium is associated with the generation of oxygen-derived free radicals. While these reactive radicals retain the ability to inflict cellular damage, they may also function in a chemotactic fashion. Evidence for this role was first put forward by Petrone *et al.* [80], who showed that generation of free radicals results in the release of a 'neutrophil chemotactic factor.' Furthermore, inhibitors of free radical production or scavengers of free radicals have been shown to decrease neutrophil infiltration [81,82]. The mechanism behind the radical-induced adhesion may be the conversion of O_2^- to H_2O_2. As mentioned previously, formation of H_2O_2 may act to stimulate a PAF–CD11/CD18-mediated adhesion. Free radical formation is likely to act as an intermediate for neutrophil chemotaxis. These radicals have been shown to activate the complement system, leading to the formation of C5a and other complement-derived factors. The ability to act as a chemoattractant and to activate the complement system suggests that free radicals are an important intermediary of the inflammatory response.

The complement cascade

The complement system has a major role in reperfusion injury in that it may have a direct effect in mediating tissue injury, as well as being responsible for orchestrating the initial sequence of events leading to the neutrophil–endothelial cell interaction. Since it was first suggested by Hill and Ward in the early 1970s [83], evidence has accumulated indicating that activation of the complement cascade during ischaemia–reperfusion contributes to tissue damage. Decomplementing an animal with cobra venom factor before the onset of myocardial infarction is associated with decreased infarct size and neutrophil infiltration [84,85]. Furthermore, components of the activated complement cascade appear in the circulation and tissues after an ischaemic event [86–89]. Rossen *et al.* [90] have reported the appearance of C1q in the plasma and ischaemic zone after reperfusion in the infarcted canine heart. The appearance of C1q correlated with the infiltration of neutrophils and the degree of the ischaemic event. This observation is supported by the appearance of C1q molecules in the circulation after a severe ischaemic event [91].

Formation and membrane insertion of the MAC is seen in the hearts of animals that have undergone experimental myocardial infarction, as well as in patients who have had a myocardial infarction. Serum analysis of post-infarct patients has shown increased concentrations of the soluble form of the MAC [86]. In addition, antibodies directed against the neoantigen of the human C5b–9 complex have been used to localize the deposition of the MAC in infarcted human myocardial tissue [88,89]. In these studies, localization of the MAC was limited to areas within the infarcted zone while the surrounding tissue was free of MAC deposition. Schafer *et al.* [88] have shown that localization of the MAC is not limited to the membrane of target cells, but may be found in the cytoplasmic regions of the cell. Thus, it is possible that components of the MAC may diffuse into the cytoplasmic space, where the complete MAC is activated by intracellular components. This observation is supported by studies showing that a number of isolated heart subcellular membranes are capable of activating the complement system, resulting in formation of the MAC [92].

The ability of complement activation to impair myocardial function has been demonstrated by Homeister *et al.* [93]. In this study, human plasma was perfused through the rabbit isolated heart, resulting in activation of the complement components found within the plasma. Activation of the complement system in this model resulted in myocardial damage, as shown by changes in biochemical and functional parameters. Further investigation has provided evidence that the MAC was the sole factor in mediating myocardial damage. Immunocytochemical studies demonstrate that the MAC is localized to both the cell membrane and intracellular components of the endothelial cell as well as the cardiac myocytes [94].

The MAC

Activation of the complement cascade may elicit tissue damage through multiple mechanisms. The primary direct action of complement is via the formation of the MAC and its insertion into the membrane of the target cell. The MAC is an amphiphilic complex composed of complement proteins C5b–9. Activation of either the classical or alternative pathways of complement is associated with the formation of the C5b–7 trimolecular complex that associates with phospholipid membranes, probably through an interaction of the membrane with C7, which contains phospholipid-binding sites [95]. Once this complex is inserted into the membrane of the target cell, proteins C8 and C9 become associated with the C5b–7 complex. The attachment of C8 to C5b–7 establishes a firm association of the complex with the membrane that may be sufficient to cause cell lysis [96]. The attachment of at least 12 to 18 C9 monomers to the C5b–8 complex within the membrane results in the formation of a circular pore, or channel, spanning the membrane. The deposition of multiple complexes on the target cell allows for the movement of water, small molecules and electrolytes across the cell membrane with ultimate loss of osmotic control, cell swelling and finally cell lysis. Nucleated cells, unlike non-nucleated cells (e.g. erythrocytes), have cellular-associated defence mechanisms that protect the cell from a limited attack by the C5b–9 complex. Thus, injury or death of nucleated cells is dependent on the intensity of the 'attack', whereby a limited number of complexes may be associated with reversible injury. On the other hand, nucleated cells may succumb to repeated and numerous insertions of the MAC. Thus, unlike the highly susceptible non-nucleated enthrocyte, irreversible damage to the nucleated cell requires 'multiple hits' by the MAC [97]. In addition to membrane damage, it has been speculated that components of complement may diffuse into the cell through the membrane channels and damage intracellular organelles. In the setting of myocardial ischaemia and reperfusion, it has been suggested that localized complement activation overwhelms the defensive mechanisms of the surrounding endothelium and cardiac myocytes, leading to cell injury or death.

In sub-lytic amounts, formation of the terminal complex acts as a potent stimulator of a number of cellular functions. The C5b–8 or C5b–9 complexes act to stimulate the release of different eicosanoids, including arachidonic acid, thromboxane B_2, and prostacyclin [79,98]. Protein synthesis is also enhanced due to MAC deposition, resulting in an increased production of cytokines, collagen and collagenases [99]. Concomitant with the increased synthesis of protein and eicosanoids is an increase in intracellular calcium and increased phospholipid turnover. Furthermore, protein kinase C and a number of G-proteins are also activated [100,101]. The direct actions of the MAC, while important in terms of inducing irreversible cell damage, are not solely responsible for cellular injury incurred during reperfusion.

Complement-mediated neutrophil function

Complement activation participates in mediating neutrophil function and recruitment into the reperfused and irreversibly damaged myocardial region.

As mentioned previously, both C3a and C5a act as chemotactic factors to recruit and activate circulating neutrophils. In addition, these cleavage products, in conjunction with C4a, alter vascular permeability by stimulating mast cells and basophils to release histamine [102,103]. The MAC also participates in initiating the inflammatory response by promoting neutrophil adhesion to the endothelium. Hattori *et al.* [104] demonstrated that human endothelial cells exposed to sub-lytic amounts of C5b–9 rapidly express the neutrophil adhesin molecule P-selectin. In addition, the MAC acts on the neutrophil itself. Although the neutrophil is provided with cell-associated defensive mechanisms, formation of a limited number of complexes can occur on the neutrophil and perhaps modify its function. The MAC may trigger the cell to release a number of different cytokines or release matrix-degrading enzymes without resulting in destruction of the neutrophil.

Activation of the complement system

While there is a substantial amount of evidence showing that complement is activated during ischaemia–reperfusion, the mechanism leading to this activation has yet to be elucidated. Under normal conditions, activation of the complement system is under rigid control, so that the low level of background activation of the complement system does not have deleterious consequences. Both erythrocytes and nucleated cells are known to possess mechanisms to protect themselves from complement attack. In addition, serum proteins (Factor I, C4-binding protein and Factor H) found in the circulation, function as inhibitors of complement activation. The presence of the cell-associated and plasma-protective mechanisms serves to localize the effects of complement within a limited area. It is likely that the events during or immediately after an ischaemic episode alter the ability of the cell to protect itself against activation of the complement cascade. This particular area has received increased attention in the hope of developing therapeutic agents to replace the inhibitory mechanisms lost during an ischaemic episode.

Complement susceptibility is increased following the damage or loss of one or more plasma proteins and membrane-associated proteins that form the regulators of complement activation. The proteins are responsible for the phenomenon of 'homologous species restriction' [105]. This term describes the ability of nucleated cells and erythrocytes to prevent lysis by complement derived from the same species. Complement receptor 1 (CR1), decay-accelerating factor and membrane cofactor protein, are membrane glycoproteins that inhibit complement activation early in the cascade (at the level of C3) [106,107]. The regulators of complement activation are found on a number of cell types, underscoring their importance in protecting tissues from endogenous attack. Two other membrane proteins, protectin (CD59, MIRL) and homologous restriction factor, act to prevent completion of the MAC within the cell membrane by preventing the binding of C8 and C9 to the C5b–7 complex [108,109]. At least one of these protective proteins, protectin, has been shown to be lost or damaged as a result of an ischaemic event [110]. Thus, ischaemia-induced loss of one or more of the regulators of complement activation would leave the cells within an infarct zone vulnerable to complement attack.

The ability of the regulatory proteins to protect the infarcted myocardium was illustrated in a study by Weisman *et al.* [111] using a soluble form of CR1 (sCR1). CR1 is an inhibitory protein found on most peripheral blood cells. The cytoplasmic and transmembrane domains of the CR1 molecule were removed, resulting in the soluble form of the molecule. When given before reperfusion, sCR1 resulted in a 44% reduction in infarct size in the rat heart, as compared with control vehicle-treated animals. Several additional reports have supported the role of sCR1 in protecting the myocardium subjected to ischaemia and reperfusion [112–114]. The protective effect of sCR1 provides additional evidence for the role of complement in myocardial injury and suggests a potential therapeutic approach for decreasing reperfusion injury.

In addition to the presence of protective proteins, nucleated cells contain defensive mechanisms that may become impaired when subjected to ischaemic stress. Nucleated cells release plasma membrane vesicles during complement attack and deposition of the MAC, suggesting that this is an important protective mechanism. Morgan [97] has shown that neutrophils remove a portion of membrane-bound MACs by internalizing or endocytosing the complex subsequent to degradation in the cell. The physical removal of the MAC is dependent on the target cell being in a condition such that these processes may be operative [115]. Cells undergoing an ischaemic event may be depleted of the necessary metabolic capabilities to carry out these types of action. The loss of defence mechanisms, coupled with the overwhelming complement-mediated attack, would leave the cell vulnerable to irreversible injury.

Formation of oxygen-derived free radicals may stimulate complement activation in both a direct and indirect manner. Free radicals may directly activate complement by converting C5 to a functionally active C5b-like form [116,117]. These observations are supported in a study by Shingu *et al.* showing that the generation of H_2O_2 by neutrophils results in complement activation. Damage to the cellular membrane may provide an indirect mechanism by which free radicals initiate activation of complement. As stated previously, damage to the membrane may take the form of denaturation of integral proteins and/or altered membrane integrity. Denaturation of protective membrane proteins impairs the ability of the cell to ward off injury via activation of the complement system. Exposure of basement membranes and subcellular organelles has been shown to activate complement [119]. Early investigations demonstrate that isolated myocardial membranes bind C1, leading to activation of the entire cascade. Furthermore, constituents on the mitochondria are able to elicit activation of the complement system. One may speculate that membrane damage due to ischaemia and/or reperfusion allows complement proteins to move into the cell or damaged organelles to move out of the cell. Regardless, the subsequent activation of complement may result in further cell injury or cell death.

Concluding remarks

It has become evident that a number of factors are involved in the cellular alterations associated with ischaemia–reperfusion injury. Oxygen-derived free radicals and the inflammatory response to injury are two of the major partici- pants in the extension of cell death beyond that resulting from the aborted ischaemic insult. Oxygen free radicals from intracellular sites in the endothe- lium and cardiac myocytes exert direct effects on cellular membranes and pro- teins. The inflammatory system, via complement activation and accumulation of neutrophils at the site of injury, has also been associated with the exten- sion of irreversible cell death. It is paradoxical that both oxygen and the inflammatory response are necessary for proper healing to occur after the completion of a myocardial infarction.

While it is tempting to discuss free radicals and the inflammatory response as separate events, it is apparent that both act in concert to extend cellular damage beyond the confines of the region injured by the period of ischaemia. The ability of free radicals to activate the complement system or damage complement regulatory proteins is a prime example of the co-opera- tive interaction. Thus, it may be speculated that inhibiting free radical forma- tion may have a modulating inhibitory effect upon complement-mediated cell injury. Inhibition of this response would not only decrease the direct effects of the MAC, but also decrease neutrophil accumulation, suppressing produc- tion of the chemotactic anaphylatoxins. It should be kept in mind, however, that a number of additional mechanisms have been offered to explain how complement is activated in response to an ischaemic insult followed by reper- fusion. Thus, it is unlikely that inhibiting oxygen-derived free radicals would serve to prevent the inflammatory response. The existence of multiple mecha- nisms for control of the inflammatory response to injury, offers a challenge for the development of pharmacological interventions directed towards the salvage of viable tissue that would otherwise be irreversibly injured during the restoration of blood flow. There is total agreement with respect to the need to restore blood flow if the ischaemic tissue is to survive. Efforts must now be directed towards reducing that component of injury associated with reper- fusion. The goal can only be achieved by a complete understanding of the basic mechanisms involved in the phenomenon by which reintroduction of oxygenated whole blood extends tissue injury beyond that resulting from the ischaemic insult. Significant progress has been achieved in a relatively short time and there is optimism that a successful outcome will be achieved. In closing, it should be appreciated that the phenomenon of reperfusion injury is not limited to the myocardium. The very same, or at least similar, mechanisms may apply to any organ or tissue that is subjected to ischaemia and subsequent reperfusion, as in the case of organ transplantation. The knowledge gained regarding the prevention of reperfusion injury, therefore has potential for wide application in clinical medicine.

Studies from the author's (BRL's) laboratory cited in this manuscript were supported by a Grant from the National Institutes of Health, Heart Lung and Blood Institute, HL-19782-15.

References

1. Topal, E.J. (1987) J. Clin. Pharmacol. **27**, 735–745
2. Jennings, R.B., Reimer, K.A. and Steenbergen, C. (1986) J. Mol. Cell. Cardiol. **18**, 769–780
3. Roberts, R., DeMello, V. and Sobel, S.E. (1976) Circulation **53** (Suppl. I), 204–206
4. Hearse, D.J., Humphrey, S.M., Nayler, W.G., Slade, A. and Border, D. (1975) J. Mol. Cell. Cardiol. **7**, 315–324
5. Zweier, J.L. (1988) J. Biol. Chem. **263**, 1353–1357
6. Kramer, J.H., Arroyo, C.M., Dickens, B.F. and Weglicki, W.B. (1987) Free Radical Biol. Med. **3**, 153–159
7. Ferrari, R., Ceconi, C., Currello, S., Guarnieri, C., Caldarera, C.M., Albertini, A. and Visioli, O. (1985) J. Mol. Cell. Cardiol. **17**, 937–945
8. Jolly, S.R., Kane, W.J., Bailie, M.B., Abrams, G.D. and Lucchesi, B.R. (1984) Circ. Res. **54**, 277–285
9. Werns, S.W., Simpson, P.J., Mickelson, J.K., Shea, M.J., Pitt, B. and Lucchesi, B.R. (1988) J. Cardiovasc. Pharmacol. **11**, 36–44
10. Tamura, Y., Chi, L., Driscoll, E.M., Hoff, P.T., Freeman, B.A., Gallagher, K.P. and Lucchesi, B.R. (1988) Circ. Res. **63**, 944–959
11. Gallagher, K.P., Buda, A.J., Pace, D., Gerren, R.A. and Schlafer, M. (1986) Circulation **73**, 1065–1076
12. Nejima, J., Knight, D.R., Fallon, J.T., Uemura, N., Manders, T., Canfield, D.R., Cohen, M.V. and Vatner, S.F. (1989) Circulation **79**, 143–153
13. Kako, K.J. (1985) Jikeikai Med. J. **32**, 609–639
14. Schaich, K.M. (1980) CRC Crit. Rev. Food Sci. Nutr. **13** (Part 3), 189–244
15. Wolff, S.P., Garner, A. and Dean, R.T. (1986) Trends Biochem. Sci. **11**, 27–31
16. Torchinsky, Y.M. (1981) in Sulfur in Proteins (Moiseevich, I., ed.; translated by Wittenberg, W.), pp. 237–277, Pergamon Press, Oxford.
17. Kako, K.J. (1987) J. Mol. Cell. Cardiol. **19**, 209–211
18. Chambers, D.E., Parks, D.A., Patterson, G., Ranjan, R., McCord, J.M., Yoshida, S., Parmley, L.F. and Downey, J.M. (1985) J. Mol. Cell. Cardiol. **17**, 145–152
19. Werns, S.W., Shea, M.J., Driscoll, E.M., Dysko, R.C., Fantone, J.C., Schork, M.A., Abrams, G.D., Pitt, B. and Lucchesi, B.R. (1986) Circulation **73**, 518–524
20. Eddy, L.J., Stewart, J.R., Jones, H.P., Engerson, T.D., McCord, J.M. and Downey, J.M. (1987) Am. J. Physiol. **253**, H709–H711
21. Muxfeldt, M. and Schaper, W. (1987) Basic Res. Cardiol. **82**, 486–492
22. Werns, S.W., Grum, C.M., Ventura, A., Hahn, R.A., Ho, P.K., Towner, R.D., Fantone, J.C., Schork, M.A. and Lucchesi, B.R. (1991) Circulation **83**, 995–1005
23. Rowe, J.T., Manson, N.H., Caplan, M. and Hess, M.L. (1983) Circ. Res. **53**, 584–591
24. Guanieri, C., Flamigni, F. and Caldarera, C.M. (1980) J. Mol. Cell. Cardiol. **12**, 797–808
25. Fishbein, M.C., Maclean, D. and Maroko, P.R. (1978) Chest **73**, 843–849
26. Jolly, S.R., Kane, W.J., Hook, B.J., Abrams, G.D., Kunkel, S.L. and Lucchesi, B.R. (1986) Am. Heart J. **112**, 682–690

27. Romson, J.L., Hook, B.G., Kunkel, S.L., Abrams, G.D., Schork, M.A. and Lucchesi, B.R. (1983) Circulation **67**, 1016–1023
28. Romson, J.L., Hook, B.G., Rigot, V.H., Schork, M.A., Swanson, D.P. and Lucchesi, B.R. (1982) Circulation **66**, 1002–1011
29. Litt, M.R., Jeramy, R.W., Weisman, H.F., Winkelstein, J.A. and Becker, L.C. (1989) Circulation **80**, 1816–1827
30. Mullane, K.M., Read, N., Salmon, J.A. and Moncada, S. (1984) J. Pharmacol. Exp. Ther. **228**, 510–522
31. Simpson, P.J., Todd, R.F. III, Fantone, J.C., Mickelson, J.K., Griffin, J.D. and Lucchesi, B.R. (1988) J. Clin. Invest. **81**, 624–629
32. Seewaldt-Becker, E., Rothlein, R., and Dammgen, J.W. (1990) in Structure and Function of Molecules Involved in Leukocyte Adhesion (Springer, T.A., Anderson, D.C., Rosenthal, A.S. and Rothlein, R., eds.), pp. 138–148, Springer-Verlag, New York.
33. Ley, K., Gaehtgens, P., Fennie, C., Singer, M.S., Laskey, L.A. and Rosen, S.D. (1991) Blood **77**, 2553–2555
34. Lasky, L.A. (1992) Science **258**, 964–969
35. Kishimoto, T.K., Warnock, R.A., Jutila, M.A., Butcher, E.C., Lane, C., Anderson, D.C. and Smith, C.W. (1991) Blood **78**, 805–811
36. Spertini, O., Kansas, G.S., Munro, J.M., Griffen, J.D. and Tedder, T.F. (1991) Nature **349**, 691–694
37. Kishimoto, T.K., Jutila, M.A., Berg, E.L. and Butcher, E.C. (1989) Science **245**, 1238–1241
38. Jutila, M.A., Rott, L., Berg, E.L. and Butcher, E.C. (1989) J. Immunol. **143**, 3318–3324
39. Sugama, Y., Tiruppathi, C., Janakidevi, K., Anderson, T.T., Fenton, J.W. II and Malik, A.B. (1992) J. Cell. Biol. **119**, 935–944
40. Patel, K.P., Zimmerman, G.A., Prescott, S.M., McEver, R.P. and McIntyre, T.M. (1991) J. Cell Biol. **112**, 749–759
41. Mulligan, M.S., Polly, M.J., Bayer, R.J., Nunn, M.F., Paulson, J.C. and Ward, P.A. (1992) J. Clin. Invest. **90**, 1600–1607
42. Garcia, J.G., Azghani, A., Callahan, K.S. and Johnson, A.R. (1988) Thromb. Res. **51**, 83–96
43. Breviario, F., Bertocchi, F., Dejana, E. and Bussolino, F. (1988) J. Immunol. **141**, 3391–3397
44. Zimmerman, G.A., Prescott, S.M. and McIntyre, T.M. (1992) Immunol. Today **13**, 93–99
45. Lorant, D.E., Patel, K.D., McIntyre, T.M., McEver, R.P., Prescott, S.M. and Zimmerman, G.A. (1991) J. Cell Biol. **115**, 223–234
46. Smith, C.W., Kishimoto, T.K., Abbass, O., Hughs, B.J., Rothlein, R., McIntire, L.V., Butcher, E., Anderson, D.C. and Abbass, O. (1991) J. Clin. Invest. **87**, 609–618
47. Beller, D.I., Springer, T.A. and Schreiber, R.D. (1982) J. Exp. Med. **156**, 1000–1009
48. Wright, S.D., Rao, P.E., van Voorhis, W.C., Craigmyle, L.S., Lida, K., Talle, M.A., Westberg, E.F., Goldstein, G. and Silverstein, S.C. (1983) Proc. Natl. Acad. Sci. U.S.A. **80**, 5699–5703
49. Simpson, P.J., Fantone, J.C., Mickelson, J.K., Gallagher, K.P., Tamura, Y., Lee, K.A., Kitzen, J.M. and Lucchesi, B.R. (1988) FASEB J. **2**, A1237 (abstract)
50. Vadas, M.A. and Gamble, J.R. (1990) Biochem. Pharmacol. **40**, 1683–1688
51. Smith, C.E., Marlin, S.D., Rothlein, R., Lawrence, M.B., McIntire, L.V. and Anderson, D.C. (1990) in Leukocyte Adhesion Molecules: Structure, Function, and Regulation (Springer, T.A. et al., eds.), pp. 170–189, Springer-Verlag, New York.
52. Luscinskas, F.W., Brock, A.F., Arnaout, M.A. and Gimbrone, M.A. Jr. (1989) J. Immunol. **142**, 2257–2263
53. Entman, M.L., Michael, L., Rossen, R.D., Dreyer, W.J., Anderson, D.C., Taylor, A.A. and Smith, C.W. (1991) FASEB J. **5**, 2529–2537
54. Gasic, A.C., McGuire, G., Krater, S., Farhood, A.I., Goldstein, M.A., Smith, C.W., Entman, M.L. and Taylor, A.A. (1991) Circulation **84**, 2154–2166
55. Lewis, M.S., Whatley, R.E., Cain, P., McIntyre, T.M., Prescott, S.M. and Zimmerman, G.A. (1988) J. Clin. Invest. **82**, 2045–2055
56. Werns, S.W. and Lucchesi, B.R. (1989) Cardiovasc. Drugs Ther. **2**, 761–769
57. Klebanoff, S.J. and Clark, R.A. (1978) in The Neutrophil, Elsevier, New York
58. Parker, C.W. (1991) Annu. Rev. Resp. Dis. **143**, S59–S60
59. Hartmann, J.R., Robinson, J.A. and Gunnar, R.M. (1977) Am. J. Cardiol. **40**, 550–555

60. Hallett, M.B., Shandell, A. and Young, H.L. (1985) Biochem. Pharmacol. **34**, 1757–1761
61. Bolli, R., Cannon, R.O., Speir, E., Goldstein, R.E. and Epstein, S.E. (1980) J. Am. Coll. Cardiol. **2**, 671–680
62. Bolli, R., Cannon, R.O., Speir, E., Goldstein, R.E. and Epstein, S.E. (1980) J. Am. Coll. Cardiol. **2**, 681–688
63. Schmid-Schonbein, G.W. and Engler, R.L. (1986) Am. J. Cardiovasc. Pathol. **1**, 15–30
64. Jerome, S.N., Smith, C.W. and Korthuis, R.J. (1993) Am. J. Physiol. **264**, H479–H483
65. Sessa, W.C. and Mullane, K.M. (1990) Br. J. Pharmacol. **99**, 553–559
66. Parker, C.W. (1984) in Fundamental Immunology (Paul, W.E. ed.), pp. 697–747, Raven Press, New York.
67. Needleman, P., Turk, J., Jakschik, B.A., Morrison, A.R. and Lefkowith, J.B. (1986) Annu. Rev. Biochem. **55**, 69–102
68. Sasaki, K., Ueno, A., Katori, M. and Kikawada, R. (1988) Cardiovasc. Res. **22**, 142–148
69. McIntyre, T.M., Zimmerman, G.A. and Prescott, S.M. (1986) Proc. Natl. Acad. Sci. U.S.A. **83**, 2204–2208
70. Lawrence, M.B. and Springer, T.A. (1991) Cell **65**, 859–873
71. Colditz, I.G. (1985) Surv. Synth. Pathol. Res. **4**, 44–68
72. Rot, A. (1992) Immunol. Today **13**, 291–294
73. Strieter, R.M, Kunkel, S.L, Showell, H.J., Remick, D.G., Phan, S.H., Ward, P.A. and Marks, R.M. (1989) Science **243**, 1467–1469
74. Schroder, J.M. and Christophers, E. (1989) J. Immunol. **142**, 244–251
75. Wen, D., Rowland, A. and Derynck, R. (1989) EMBO J. **8**, 1761–1766
76. Huber, A.R., Kunkel, S.L., Todd, R.F. III and Weiss, S.J. (1991) Science **254**, 99–102
77. Detmers, P.A., Lo, S.K., Olsen-Egbert, E., Walz, A., Beggiolini, M. and Cohn, Z.A. (1990) J. Exp. Med. **171**, 1155–1162
78. Smith, W.B., Gamble, J.R., Clark-Lewis, I. and Vadas, M.A. (1993) Immunology **78**, 491–497
79. Imagawa, D.K., Osifchin, N.E., Paznekas, W.A., Shin, M.L. and Mayer, M.M. (1983) Proc. Natl. Acad. Sci. U.S.A. **80**, 6647–6651
80. Petrone, W.F., English, D.K., Wong, K. and McCord, J.M. (1980) Proc. Natl. Acad. Sci. U.S.A. **77**, 1159–1169
81. Granger, D.N. (1988) Am. J. Physiol. **255**, H1269–H1275
82. Inauen, W., Granger, D.N., Meininger, C.J., Schelling, M.E., Ganger, H.J. and Kvietys, P.R. (1990) Am. J. Physiol. **259**, H925–H931
83. Hill, J.H. and Ward, P.A. (1971) J. Exp. Med. **133**, 885–900
84. Maroko, P.R., Carpenter, C.B., Chiareillo, M., Fishbein, M.C., Radvany, P., Knostman, J.D. and Hale, S.L. (1978) J. Clin. Invest. **61**, 661–670
85. Crawford, M.H., Grover, F.L., Kolb, W.P., McMahan, A., OÚaRourke, R.A., McManus, L.M. and Pinckard, R.N. (1988) Circulation **78**, 1449–1458
86. Langlois, P.F. and Gawryl, M.S. (1988) Atherosclerosis **70**, 95–105
87. Yasuda, M., Takeuchi, K., Hiruma, M., Iida, H., Tahara, A., Itagane, H., Toda, I., Akioka, K., Teragaki, M., Oku, H., et al. (1990) Circulation **81**, 156–163
88. Schafer, H., Mathey, D., Hugo, F. and Bhakdi, S. (1986) J. Immunol. **137**, 1945–1949
89. Rus, H.G., Niculescu, F. and Vlaicu, R. (1987) Immunol. Lett. **16**, 15–20
90. Rossen, R.D., Swain, J.L., Michael, L.H., Weakley, S., Giannini, E. and Entman, M.L. (1985) Circ. Res. **57**, 119–130
91. Rossen, R.D., Michael, L.H., Kagiyama, A., Savage, H.E., Hanson, G., Reisberg, M.A., Moake, J.N., Kim, S.H., Self, D. and Weakley, S. (1988) Circ. Res. **62**, 572–584
92. Pinckard, R.N., Olson, M.S., Kelley, R.E., Detter, D.H., Palmer, J.D., OÚaRourke, R.A. and Goldfein, S. (1973) J. Immunol. **110**, 1376–1382
93. Homeister, J.W., Satoh, P. and Lucchesi, B.R. (1992) Circ. Res. **71**, 303–319
94. Homeister, J.W., Satoh, P.S., Kilgore, K.S. and Lucchesi, B.R. (1993) J. Immunol. **150**, 1055–1064
95. Atkinson, J.P. and Liszewski, M.K. (1991) in Immunology (Schwartz, B.D., ed.), pp. 111–131, Scope Publications, Kalamazoo, Michigan, U.S.A.
96. Morgan, B.P. (1990) in Complement: Clinical Aspects and Relevence to Disease (Morgan, B.P., ed.), pp. 1–35, Academic Press, San Diego.

97. Morgan, B.P. (1989) Biochem. J. **264**, 1–14
98. Hansch, G.M., Seitz, M., Martinotti, G., Betz, M., Rauterberg, E.W. and Gemsa, D. (1984) J. Immunol. **133**, 2145–2150
99. Klostermann, M., Schols, M. and Hansch, G.M. (1992) Immunobiology **184**, 433 (abstract)
100. Betz, M., Seitz, M. and Hansch, G.M. (1987) Int. Arch. Allergy Appl. Immunol. **8**, 313–316
101. Niculescu, F., Lang, T., Rus, H. and Shin, M.L. (1991) Complement Inflammation **8**, 199 (abstract)
102. Vogt, W. (1986) Complement **3**, 177–188
103. Hugli, T.E. (1983) in Biological Response Mediators and Modulators (August, J.T., ed.), pp. 99–116, Academic Press, New York.
104. Hattori, R., Hamilton, K.K., McEver, R.P. and Sims, P.J. (1989) J. Biol. Chem. **264**, 9053–9060
105. Hansch, G.M., Hammer, C.H., Vanguri, P. and Shin, M.L. (1981) Proc. Natl. Acad. Sci. U.S.A. **78**, 5118–5121
106. Lublin, D.M. and Atkinson, J.P. (1989) Annu. Rev. Immunol. **7**, 35–59
107. Cole, J., Haisly, G.A., Dykman, T.R., MacDemott, R.P. and Atkinson, J.B. (1985) Proc. Natl. Acad. Sci. U.S.A. **83**, 859–864
108. Sugita, Y., Nakano, Y. and Tomita, M. (1988) J. Biochem. (Tokyo) **104**, 633–637
109. Davies, A., Simmons, D.L., Hale, G., Harrison, R.A., Tighe, H., Lachmann, P.J. and Waldmann, H. (1989) J. Exp. Med. **170**, 637–654
110. Vakeva, A., Laurila, P. and Meri, S. (1992) Lab. Invest. **67**, 608–616
111. Weisman, H.F., Bartow, T., Leppo, M.K., Marsh, H.C. Jr, Carson, G.R., Concino, M.F., Boyle, M.P., Roux, K.H., Weisfeldt, M.L. and Fearon, D.T. (1990) Science **249**, 146–151
112. Shandelya, S., Fearon, D., Weisfeldt, M. and Zweier, J. (1991) Circulation **84** (Suppl II), II-83 (abstract)
113. Smith, E.F. III, DiMartino, M.J., Davis, P.A., Egan, J.W., Griswold, D.E., Hilleglass, L.M., Fong, K.-L., Brown, K.S. and Crysler, C.S. (1991) Circulation **84** (Suppl II), II-83 (abstract)
114. Shin, M.L. and Carney, D. (1988) Prog. Allergy **40**, 44–81
115. Ohanian, S.H. and Schlager, S.I. (1981) Crit. Rev. Immunol. **1**, 165–209
116. Vogt, W., von Zabern, I., Hesse, D., Nolte, R. and Haller, Y. (1986) Immunol. Lett. **14**, 209–215
117. Vogt, W., Damerau, B., von Zabern, I., Nolte, R. and Brunahl, D. (1989) Mol. Immunol. **26**, 1133–1142
118. Shingu, M., Nonaka, S., Nishimukai, H., Nobunaga, M., Kitamura, H. and Tomo-Oka, K. (1992) Clin. Exp. Immunol. **90**, 72–78
119. Williams, J.D., Czop, J.K., Abrahamson, D.R., Davies, M. and Austen, K.F. (1984) J. Immunol. **133**, 394–399

Index